Healing
for the
Age of Enlightenment

BALANCED NUTRITION
VITA FLEX
COLOR THERAPY

by
STANLEY BURROUGHS

For Your Information

Burroughs Books
3702 S. Virginia St.
Ste. # G-12 Box 346
Reno, NV 89502-6030
Fax # 1-775-972-4899

Healing for the Age of Enlightenment

$12.00

Shipping & Handling — Add $1.50

plus .75 for each additional book shipped

**Make Check or Money Order Payable
To: Burroughs Books**

 Visa/MasterCard accepted

Please include expiration date

Sixth Edition

Burroughs Books
3702 S. Virginia St.
Ste. # G-12 Box 346
Reno, NV 89502-6030
Fax # 1-775-972-4899
ISBN # 0-9639262-1-7

"A WINNING COMBINATION"

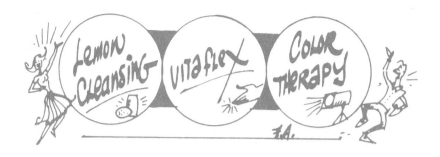

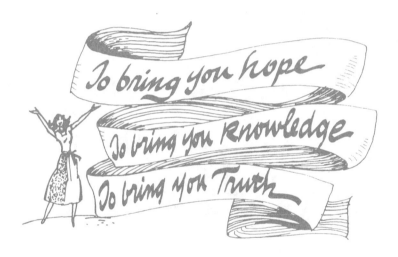

I present this book so that you can help yourself and others. Make the most of this work and know that it is the finest of knowledge in healing.

"Let no man refuse to listen and be healed lest he bring misery, pain and suffering to those who look and depend on him for help and guidance."

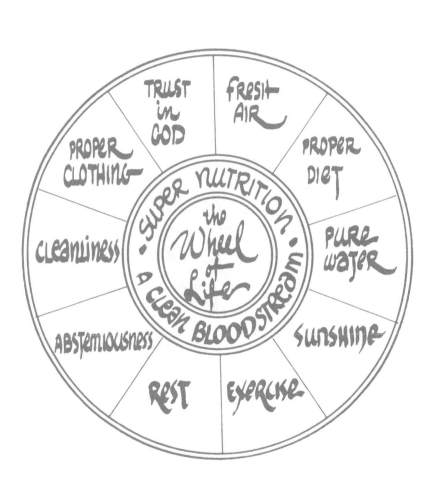

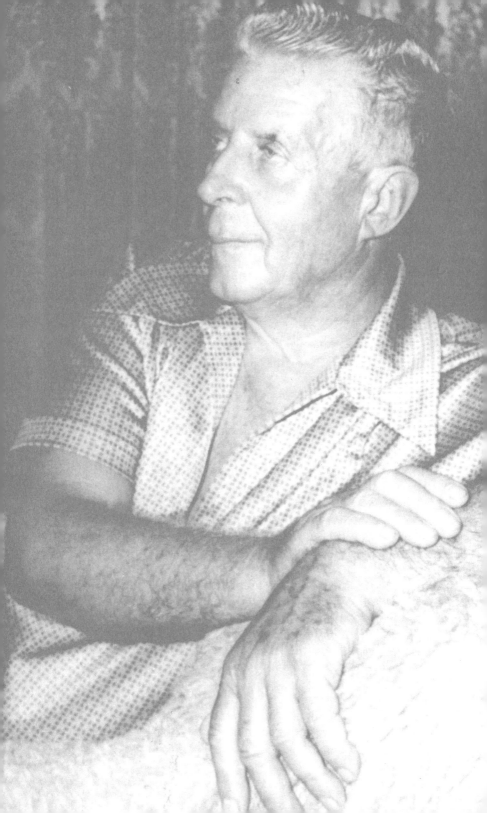

The Famous Germ and Virus Gang

A CURE FOR WHICH THERE WAS NO KNOWN DISEASE

Medicine is constantly researching endlessly for a cure for all diseases but always coming up empty handed.

Medicine could be the only one who could be so ignorant or so corrupt as to convince the government to pay 150 million dollars for a cure for a disease that never existed. This cure was administered to millions of victims causing a variety of other diseases that still have no cure available.

With all the failures to find a cure for a variety of diseases, medicine finally hit the jackpot, they found a cure for a disease that existed only in a confused mind — the "Swine flu."

The false cure for the non existant Swine flu became the worst nightmare of criminal action that should have been prosecuted as a crime of the century but they got away without any form of charges or discreditment.

The disease never materialized to either the millions who took the cure or to the many more millions who never took it but the side effects from the cure were most devastating to the victims. Why was no legal action taken against the offenders?

About The Author

Stanley Burroughs, now deceased, developed a successful system which has already revolutionized the entire understanding of the art of healing.

It is a brilliant and fresh approach to healing in its simplest form.

He has searched tirelessly, throughout the many years, to find these natural laws of healing. He has simplified and clarified them for fast and accurate results. The work is easy to understand and use as an aid to find complete freedom and release from any and all kinds of illnesses regardless of by what name they may be called.

These techniques and principles do not depend on faith, belief or special religious rituals.

This system proves, by actual results, that there is absolutely no need for further expenditures of millions of dollars for useless and time consuming research to find the cause and correction of any present or future variety of diseases. The complete answers are already here.

The professions and the public alike are strongly invited to make any and all possible tests of the work. If this is done honestly and with the best interests of the public in mind every part of the work will be found accurate and outstanding as the highest form of the healing arts.

It is a system of automatic precision which can eliminate the many human errors which can and do occur with the present awkward, complicated and ever more costly methods.

This system accepts no limitations as to the ability of the body to heal itself.

Acknowledgments

I wish to acknowledge the constant presence and inspiration from the Universal Mind which has made it possible for me to bring to the healing world of misinformation and confusion the many simple rules of healing that govern and control all phases of the healing arts.

I wish to take this opportunity to thank you, all of my wonderful friends throughout the world, for it is you who have made it possible for me to publish this book. Without you, and your eagerness for a more healthful and creative life, I could never have had the opportunity, nor have developed the ability, to prove that this system really works better than any other method.

My undying gratitude goes to those who have so generously offered their precious time, abilities, materials and equipment to help put this book in a most presentable form.

My dear Wife, Louise, who has now passed on, deserves much credit as a critic offering advice and encouragement through many dificult years because she believed this system had great merit, need and universal appeal. Many weeks of typing and retyping helped me meet a very close deadline.

Carol Rawlings' most generous offer of time for the final typing of many copies has been most invaluable. Her husband, Robert, was one of the supposedly incurable cases of a serious illness – now made whole because of this work.

Ralph Odom, with his delightful way with words, has done so much to improve the quality and understanding of this volume.

Rama Devi added her much needed abilities for the greatest part of the photography.

William C. Finley, Professor and accomplished student in Sanskrit has generously offered a much needed article on Yoga. This accurate and authentic report (translation) of a very ancient art as an aid to many forms of healing has added so much knowledge and inspiration to millions of people for centuries.

Robert P. Sandberg, M.S., has helped add much needed information on the biochemistry of nutrition and color.

Foreword

The purpose of this book is to bring to its readers a knowledge and a way of living which, in the experience of the author, has consistently demonstrated itself superior in every way to every other system in popular use today.

The work is based on results occurring over a period of more than fifty years of working with patients of virtually every known disease and disorder from simple physical and mental cases to the more difficult and supposedly terminal conditions. This volume is thus a report of actually experienced and consistent results; it is not mere theory or guesswork.

To be complete, a healing system must be able to encompass the entire range of human experience—physical, mental, and spiritual. Any system which denies or ignores any aspect of this trinity fails in its attempt to heal to the same extent that it denies any part or parts of the whole.

This book deals primarily with well-defined, simple, basic laws which relate to cleansing, structural changes, and natural healing. Although it may appear at first glance to deal only with the physical, further depth and understanding will reveal that it also makes use of mental and spiritual laws and that its author views health as an interrelated totality involving the entire person.

This system makes the most difficult procedures in healing seem so simple, so easy and so effective.

THE HUMAN COMPUTER

A woman becomes pregnant and immediately the divine intelligence within takes over and a baby is formed. The woman has no control as to where the different parts are placed. It is all directed automatically by the divine computer within the mother and the newly developing mortal.

To many people , God seems so far away. If so who did the moving?

This entire book is based on the automatic computer action in the body.

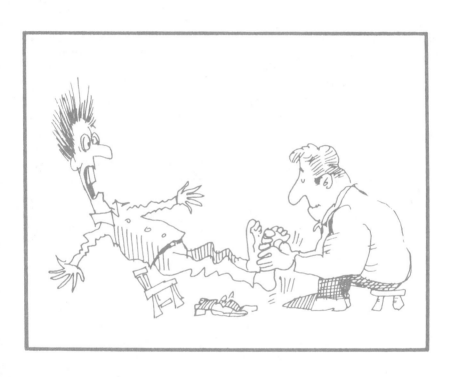

Contents

Introduction

All orthodox publicly accepted systems of healing have limitations. These limitations exist largely because of the lack of understanding of the interrelatedness of all functions of the human body.

Healing arts involving bodily manipulations — Chiropractic, Osteopathy, exercises, yoga, and traditional forms of massage — are limited by their incomplete theories and applications. In the healing arts, involving the administering of various types of medication, limitations similarly exist because of a partial understanding of interrelated bodily functions. In the effort to overcome these limitations many unnatural, synthetic, and actually destructive practices have emerged.

There are many elements to the field of physical healing. Human beings have a physical body and it must be used and developed to maintain proper circulation and performance of bodily functions. An inactive life can only bring on unfavorable conditions. Exercise is thus a basic requirement for development and healing of the physical body. This includes a wide range of activities; dancing, acrobatics, games, water sports, and many track and field events can develop skills that are of tremendous benefit. A large variety of gymnasium sports and exercises are of great value. Physical labor should also be regarded as a part of healing — relief and healing often results from gainful labor. One of the finest systems of physical well-being, if properly taught, is the regular practice of yoga; stretching exercises. Hatha Yoga is tops in the field.

A well-trained masseur can perform what sometimes seem like miracles in a most pleasant way by bringing relief to tired, sore, pained and aching muscles and joints. Massage relaxes tension, increases circulation, loosens congestions, and stimulates all the organs and cells of the body. This system is the oldest form of healing known to man and still today is one of the most effective ways to better health. Included in scientific massage are the many forms of reflex massage which, when properly used, can produce numerous structural changes or corrections and aid in removing pressures which slow down or depress normal activities in all body functions. Steam baths, frequently used in conjunction with massage and physical exercises, are of tremendous benefit as an aid to natural healing and living. The finest of reflex massage will be completely explained in this book.

Another form of specialized physical healing which has come to us down through the ages is the use of herbs. Their properties or abilities are mainly to supply needed elements which may be missing as the result of a faulty diet. Some herbs have been used to loosen congestion, others to aid in the elimination of poisons from the body.

With the increased use of these herbs there naturally developed specialists desiring to increase their use by packaging and promoting them as forms of medicine. As medicines thus increased, specialized laboratories in more recent times began isolating the various ingredients of the herbs in an effort to make them more potent. As this occurred, many of the balancing effects of the herbs disappeared and unpleasant side effects began to take place. The drug companies then began to produce the elements found in herbs synthetically from chemicals. Stronger and stronger drugs were produced with ever-increasing and more dangerous side effects until the entire situation became a compli-cated nightmare of "kill or cure" proportions!

Poisons, drugs, and chemotherapy are a part of these destructive forces. When these did not properly work, psychology and psychiatry became a part of medical practice in an effort to overcome the limitations which continue to exist. Many of these efforts to reduce the limitations have come from outside the medical field and gradually, one by one, are being reluntantly accepted as part of the healing profession. (Acupunc-ture is a recent case in point.)

Diagnosis and prescribing became boundless and extreme in the attempt to apply substances designed to destroy what was believed to be the causes of man's diseases. In spite of increasing medication, however, diseases have actually increased . . . and so have the many forms of medication.

Hundreds of names have been given to a huge variety of conditions (diseases) until volumes are needed to catalogue all of the procedures for diagnosis and treatment.

Still the mystery of disease remained unsolved and another solution automatically developed. Gradually specialists emerged whose theory was that if they couldn't stop the onslaught of disease by medication, then they would cut out the diseased parts of the body to solve the problem. But they still continued medication . . . nothing else to do since they must kill those pesky germs which were presumed to be the major cause of illness.

Next solution: research. Has it been successful? Foundations and government appropriated millions of dollars. More and more groups were formed for disease research. More millions poured in as more promises were given: "Success is just around the corner," "give till it hurts," "there will soon be a breakthrough." The money came in . . . but the breakthrough just didn't come through. Those pesky little germs and viruses just wouldn't give up their secrets!

Could it be that the medics had been spending so much time and money looking for the germs, and the chemicals to destroy them, that they never had time to find the disease? Perhaps the germs were not the cause after all, but the results. Perhaps the disease came first and then the germs. Perhaps the germs even aided in getting rid of the disease.

Some individuals began working on this principle and came up with all the answers without collecting or spending millions of other peoples' money. The truth was simple. The rules were simple. Incorrect nutrition was the underlying cause. Bad food caused congestion and toxic conditions — which in turn caused malfunction of the cells and organs and produced overall deficiencies. To supply these dificiencies another group discovered and isolated first "vitamins," then minerals (natural ingredients of foods, of course), put them in tablet and liquid form and packaged them in bottles. We became a nation of "pill pushers." There was even a dream that one day every need would be supplied by a pill or group of pills! Research has not completely determined just how and what the body really needs and how it uses it despite the fact that tremendous strides have been made in vitamin and mineral research. Many conclusions have resulted, such as the five classifications of foods which are needed daily and a certain number of essential vitamins. With all this research, however, the limitations have still remained.

There are wide differences of opinion among the "experts" and in the meantime people continue to be sick, concluding that further research must be what is necessary.

To find the simple answers, we need only look to nature and become aware of the simple laws involved.

A mind and power greater than ours has already set up laws and plans which work. We have only to work knowingly with these laws and patterns and our endless search for health is over. It is only when man decides he knows more than God, and works contrary to the way He has established, that man becomes sick. This is neither religious fanaticism nor pious platitude — just the plain fact discoverable by anyone open and willing to discover it: working in conformity with the laws of nature results in health; violating these laws results in illness.

The body does not stumble along blindly. Rather, it is well-controlled and organized to function automatically according to precise and accurate plans. Any healing approach which does not include this understanding fails in its ability to utilize the fullness of the body's potentials. Operations, drugs, unnatural medicine, shots, and antibiotics can never begin to compete with the complex yet simple automatic laws of creative healing.

"Drugs" are essentially chemicals designed to alter the natural behavior of cells and various bodily processes. The presumption is that our cells are functioning badly and that these chemicals will correct their undesirable behavior. But chemical alteration of bodily processes can be extremely harmful, and therefore we are told not to take them except when prescribed or administered by a licensed practitioner. The average person is not even allowed to purchase most of these drugs without a prescription, so dangerous are they considered to be!

When any person (or group, be it ever so prestigious!) attempts to put a man-made system above God and His healing plan, the results are bound to be failure, even disaster.

Licensed medical practitioners alone are permitted legally to prescribe a large variety of essentially destructive drugs to anyone who comes for help. Does this permission imply that these practitioners are so wise that they can know all of the effects of these drugs upon each person for whom they are prescribed? Does it suggest that they are above the law and that a dangerous drug suddenly becomes safe because the doctor prescribes it? Can he make an unsafe drug safe? Does he have the God-given powers greater than the powers of the "poisons"? (Think about it. Isn't this what they are — poisons?) How can he make potentially death dealing drugs suddenly harmless and healing at the same time?

The facts are that nothing the doctor can do will change the true nature of drugs and poisons. They remain the same regardless of how advanced toward the Divine he may consider himself to be. **All forms of medication have their dangerous side effects.**

If there were no other way, then the hope of possible correction might be worth taking such dangerous risks. But since there are other ways, truly this archaic and destructive system has no justifiable reason for further use. Very likely the reader has discovered in his own experience that once reliance on the drug way has begun, rarely can it be stopped or the healing completed. The treatment goes on and on and the dosage increases as the regular dose becomes less and less effective to relieve the suffering. Only temporary relief is in sight — the pain is still there and the diseased condition remains. We are told we must "learn to live with our diseases."

The reluctance of the medical profession to seek out and exhaust the possibilities of natural methods has been the strongest incentive to encourage other people to investigate this field. Surely the simple, natural, and easy way is always the best — particularly since it works!

As alternative healing methods emerged the medical practitioners were growing in power, and their leaders realized that laws must be made to protect them from competition. Laws were indeed enacted, but competition came anyway.

Thousands of sufferers found that they needed more than medicine had to offer.It was their search and need which led to the development of other systems. Those utilyzing alternative methods of healing were prosecuted as frauds even though they helped many people solve their health problems. Even licensed medical practitioners were prosecuted for using methods not approved by their profession. The more they helped people, the more they were prosecuted. People continued to search out and go to other systems to find the help they needed because medicine did not give them what they wanted. Even though organized medicine used the laws to defeat competition, the people continued going to other systems. They knew what they wanted and would not be denied.

Had the medical profession been right, competent to heal and give all the answers, then there would be no need or place for competition.

The medical profession has constantly used placebos that have little or no value in the healing process. The Food and Drug Administration has said repeatedly that a large proportion of the drugs used by doctors have little or no ability to heal the conditions for which they are used. Is not the irresponsible use of drugs (or placebos) the real fraud? Does it become legal — or moral — to use drugs just because one has a license to practice medicine? A fraud is a fraud, regardless of who perpetrates it, particularly when the patient is paying a high price for a useless product.

Another aspect of medical practice, noted briefly previously, consists of those doctors who began to experiment with the possibility of healing by cutting out diseased or affected parts. This seemed a quick and practical solution to many problems. Specialization gradually developed and highly skilled surgeons became the elite in the medical field. From apparent, and sometimes dramatic, "successes" (i.e., heart transplants — how successful really?), came inflated egos and distorted thinking that all human malfunctions could be solved by cutting in and cutting something or anything out. It became a form of mania. They even had to operate to see if they needed to operate! The end results, or the side effects, of the operation were rarely considered; the doctor had done his job well and what happened after that was not his concern. "The operation was a success but the patient died!" The operation was successful and the mere fact that the victim might be left crippled, maimed, and miserable was not considered either before or after the operation. If the first operation was not enough and further changes were necessary — in the doctor's opinion — then a second or a third were often done.

In many cases there was still a problem, or other problems or side effects, that had no answers. This was lamentable but unavoidable. The surgeon had done his job and the patient must live with it. Drugs and medication, frequently more and more potent narcotics, were offered as relief.

There is a medical "ethic" that justifies any wrongdoing in the guise of promoting health. This protection is too often used as a shield for the exposure of mistakes that can sometimes be most devastating for a patient's entire life. The code protects one; the supposed ends justify the means by which the irreparable damage takes place.

In various ways the statement has often been made that even if there is a simpler, easier, and less expensive way — even a less destructive way — because the doctor is a surgeon, naturally he will do it with surgery. After all, this is his special skill — he earns his living by it!

In similar situations, where severe or near terminal situations exist, even though simple natural corrections can be made very quickly, only the accepted methods will be allowed. Why can't these accepted methods be changed? What has to be done to make the changes? Why are those who have the answers not even permitted to demonstrate them? How reminiscent of Galileo in an earlier day inviting the authorities to just look through his telescope and discover for themselves the truth of his teachings! — they wouldn't even look for their minds were made up to the contrary.

Just because a person has a degree and a license it should not permit him to make the many direct and indirect errors that have and will continue to occur throughout the history of the medical profession.

Many successful malpractice suits have raised the cost of medical insurance so high that some doctors have ceased to practice. Continued mistakes and costly errors may soon destroy the profession. The situation must be corrected by investigating and wholeheartedly accepting the knowledge and experience of the many better methods now in use.

Recently some changes have indeed occurred. A few of the more conscientious and dedicated of the healing professions are beginning to look further into the natural forms of healing to minimize their limitations. As usual, they are being highly criticized, condemned, and persecuted for their efforts. The change has come and will continue by leaps and bounds because the people are demanding it in ever-increasing volume. The limitations of the accepted systems must be done away with.

To meet the demand for simpler and more complete answers, many new ideas have entered the healing arena of the Western World. Acupuncture, Shiatsu, Do'in, increased activity in massage, Rolfing, expansion in the application of Yoga, awareness of natural nutrition, and many more have gradually, but surely produced, among thoughtful people, an enlarged conception of the possibilities of what can be further achieved to reduce existing limitations.

Various types of "mind control," such as Scientology, Science of Mind, and EST have been heavily promoted. The apparent achievements of these mind development techniques make us further realize that there are still limitations to overcome. Even though down through the centuries psychic and spiritual healing have always existed, there have also been limitations to their practice.

These limitations exist in all separate fields because of the lack of understanding that man is all of these things — body-mind-spirit — and not merely one or another part. When you can bring all of these systems together in a simplified form, combining all of the natural laws pertaining to every phase of being, suddenly limitations disappear. Limitations that continue to exist do so because of the limited understanding of the person or persons involved and not because of the laws involved. As we gradually erase these mis-understandings from these persons, then their limitations decrease and disappear. As we put these complete laws into action to bring about healing, all forms of errors and mistakes and side effects disappear and only positive results occur. And only when they work, and work without error, may they be called true and right.

As a complete understanding of this healing principle is universally accepted, then all phases of disease with its suffering, aches and pains, and maladjustments will no longer exist. As man understands and works knowingly with all the laws of health and their creative forces, then he no longer has to study and learn the many complications and forms of diseases. The forms of disease are different, as the leaves on the tree are all different, yet are all leaves. We don't have to know the intricate laws involved, nor do we need to know all the intricate laws in the various principles of healing and perfect health. We only need to know how to put these into action and our Creator does the rest.

The simplicity, completeness, and accuracy of the unfolding natural healing methods are overwhelming. It is hard for the ordinary mind to realize that regardless of whether we understand them or not, the methods work, and after all, this is the important point. As we put these laws into action and make them work, then little by little we are given the answers as to why they work, and gradually a completeness eliminates all limitations — except as our Creator possibly sees a need for temporary limitations, which can later be eliminated.

Even though a great deal of this knowledge seems new and revolutionary to many people, actually it has long existed and has merely been waiting for someone in our present time to bring it out into the open and make it useful to the general public. This is not an attempt to bring something new into the world, but rather to revive the ageless and make it possible for these simple laws to be used to the greatest advantage.

Many of the principles that are presented in this book may be completely contrary to everything you have believed and studied. Regardless of whether you believe them or not, it does not alter the fact that they may be true. Before you attempt to argue or deny these facts, test them as given to you and use them until you have proven them either right or wrong. Every statement and bit of information given is the accumulation of years of experience, research, and results — therefore given as facts. Make these tests and be completely satisfied that you, too, can experience the same results. At no point will any attempt be made to confuse you with theories that cannot be proven or that will not prove themselves to be right. There is no desire to give you complications, or words that have little meaning, or "double talk" without clarity. Simplicity and accuracy will be the theme through the entire book.

This three fold system accepts no limitations as to the ability of the human body to heal itself.

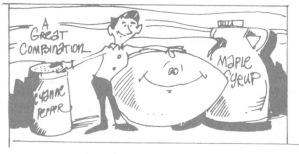

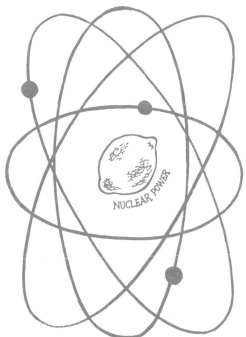

SEE, THE LEMON IS IMPORTANT

CHAPTER I

The Master Cleanser

For the novice and the advanced student alike, **cleansing** is basic for the elimination of every kind of disease. The purpose of this book is to simplify the cause and the correction of all disorders, regardless of the name or names. As we eliminate and correct one disease, we correct them all, for every disease is corrected by the same process of building positive good health.

At last the basic cause of disease is no longer a mystery. The basic cause is the habits of improper diet, inadequate exercise, negative mental attitudes, and lack of spiritual attunement which combine to produce toxic conditions and malfunction of our bodies. The elimination of the cause of illness is the obvious and only way to healing and health. The elimination of the habits that cause illness is done through the positive approach of developing proper habits that cause health combined with corrective techniques that remove the ill effects of our former incorrect ways. This book details the corrective techniques and proper habits for achieving and maintaining good health, thus releasing our potential for truly **living creatively**.

The following program has been tested and approved since 1940 in all sections of the world as the most successful of any diet of its type. **Nothing** can compare with its positive approach toward perfection in the cleansing and healing field. Nothing can compare with its rapidity and completeness. It is superior in every way as a reducing and body conditioning diet.

When we finally become sick of being sick, then we are ready to learn the truth and the truth shall set us free. This diet will prove that no one needs to live with his diseases. Lifetime freedom from disease can become a reality.

As the originator of this superior diet, I humbly and yet proudly offer it to you, confident that you will receive vigorous good health from its use.

A Word About "Epidemics" and "Germ-Caused" Diseases

Throughout the history of man, there have been constant epidemics of many diseases. Little has been known or understood as to why these things happen. (In earlier times they were thought variously to be the work of the devil, punishment from God, or poisoning of the water supply by an enemy). In recent times it has been believed that these many diseases are contagious and that germs have spread them. This belief has created a monster as the medical field has steadily found stronger and more potent drugs, poisons, and antibiotics in their constant effort to destroy what they believe to be the cause. A large variety of vaccines and antitoxins have been developed because of the belief in a large variety of bacteria and viruses.

Always the belief is that we must kill these forms of life in order to keep us free from disease. Yet, in spite of massive research, manufacturing, and wide use of these items, mankind still goes on suffering from an ever-increasing variety of disease and disorders with no let up in sight.

Disease, old age, and death are the result of accumulated poisons and congestions throughout the entire body. These toxins become crystallized and hardened, settling around the joints, in the muscles, and throughout the billions of cells all over the body.

It is presumed by orthodox medicine that we have a perfectly healthy body until something, such as germs or viruses, comes along to destroy it, whereas actually the building material for the organs and cells is defective and thus they are inferior or diseased.

Lumps and growths are formed all over the body as storage spots for unusable and accumulated waste products, especially in the lymphatic glands. These accumulations depress and deteriorate in varied degrees, causing degeneration and decay. The liver, spleen, colon, stomach, heart, and our other organs, glands, and cells come in for their share of accumulations, thus impairing their natural action.

These growths and lumps appear to us as forms of fungi. Their spread and growth is dependent on the unusuable waste material throughout the body. As the deterioration continues, our growths increase in size to take care of the situation. Fungi absorb the poisons and try to take the inferior material from the organs. This is a part of Nature's plan to rid the body of our diseases. When we stop feeding these fungi and cleanse our system, we stop their development and spread; then they dissolve or break up and pass from the body. They will not feed on healthy tissue. There is a simple set of laws which explains this action. Nature never produces anything it does not need and it never keeps anything it does not use. All unused material or waste is broken down by bacteria action into a form that can be used over again or eliminated from the body. All weak and deficient cells, caused from improper nutrition will also be broken down and eliminated from the body.

We spend a good portion of our lives accumulating these diseases and we spend the rest of our lives attempting to get rid of them — or die in the effort!

The incorrect understanding of the above truths has led uncivilized and civilized nations alike to search for some magic "cure" in all kinds of charms, witchcraft, and unlimited kinds of obnoxious poisons and

2

drugs. In general, they are worse than useless because they cannot possibly eliminate the cause of any disease. They can only add more misery and suffering and shorten one's life still further. It has been reported in many books and magazine articles that many new diseases and disorders have been created by orthodox and hospital methods.

As we continue to search for more and more magic "cures" we become more and more involved with complicated varieties of disease. A simple understanding and action has always proved to be the best to eliminate our negative actions and reactions.

Germs and viruses do not and cannot cause any of our diseases, so we have no need for finding various kinds of poisons to destroy them. **In fact, man will never find a poison or group of poisons strong enough to destroy all the billions upon billions of these germs without destroying himself at the same time.**

These germs are our friends, there are no bad ones, and if given a chance will break up and consume these large amounts of waste matter and assist us in eliminating them from the body. These germs and viruses exist in excess only when we provide a breeding ground in which they can multiply. Germs and viruses are in the body to help break down waste material and can do no harm to healthy tissues.

Do you think that if an insignificant, microscopic microbe can appear and make you sick when you were well and strong, that you have any possibility of getting strong enough to throw them off at any time thereafter? Do you think that any destructive poisons can make it possible for you to get well any faster?

All diseases, regardless of their names, come within this understanding as only varied expressions of the one disease of **toxemia.**

As noted earlier, we are constantly told that the medical researchers are about to make a big breakthrough and finally conquer all our diseases. This breakthrough will never happen until their false approach to science is replaced by the natural science of the secret of life energy and its creative action within us. Through an open-minded approach to the truth about the life force or energy, we can know the underlying facts behind epidemics and eliminate their cause.

Basically, all of our diseases are created by ourselves because we have never taken the time to discover the true foods meant for man's use. We can create healthy bodies by using the right foods and eliminating highly toxic and mucus-forming foods.

As you learn more about nutrition you will become aware of the many foods that cause excess mucus in our bodies and then realize that this condition becomes the breeding ground for all kinds of germs.

We know that throughout nature everything moves in cycles, constantly changing, constantly cleaning out the old and building the new. Consequently, as a person reaches the "point of no return," a point where his accumulations have reached the limit of what the body can

3

tolerate, then a rapid change takes place or he dies. The cycle has come to the point where a good house cleaning must be started, and one of nature's most effective methods is to start loosening and eliminating these poisons with bacteria action. As this action progresses, we become sick and feverish; large amounts of mucus are eliminated; diarrhea increases the discharge of waste material; and all of our resources go into action to clean us out as fast as possible to prevent these poisons from killing us. When this happens do not panic and resort to the unnatural action of drugs and antibiotics which can only defeat natures laws. The drugs stop the natural changes by suppressing the cleansing action and stores the poisons in the body to cause future problems.

If we know these danger signals and engage our abilities in their maximum effort, we can survive the ordeal and live a normal life until further accumulations trigger another life change. However, the logical procedure is **to prevent these accumulations from forming in the first place** — then we have no need for the discomfort of the severe cleansing process.

As the above conditons happen to more and more people at the same time an "epidemic" is set in motion. Very often an epidemic occurs after holiday feasting. Even the very best of foods in excess can create problems. If only a sufficient amount of good food is consumed, a severe cleansing-illness-will not be required as the normal operation of the body will then be adequate.

Deficiencies do exist, primarily because of improper diet and improper assimilation. These deficiencies also produce toxins because of the deterioration of the cells. So we still have only one disease, and with one simple process we can eliminate all so-called diseases of whatever name. As we expel the disease-producing toxins from our bodies, we must also restore the deficiencies. Thus, a cleansing diet **must also include proper material for building as the waste material is eliminated.**

There is still one more factor involved to make the total process completely understandable. Since germs do not cause our disorders, there must be another logical reason for the triggering of an epidemic. This is a matter of simple "vibration." The better the physical and mental condition a person is in, the higher becomes his vibration, but as he steadily becomes clogged with more and more waste matter, his vibration goes constantly downward until he is ready and in need of a change. If he then comes in contact with one or more who have already started the cleansing process, he picks up the vibration of change and all his functions are triggered into the same action. This can happen to any size group of people in similar condition, and then an epidemic is on its way. The person with a toxic free body and undisturbed mind is the one unaffected by the epidemic.

Perhaps it is a good thing that Medicine and Nature never got together – Nature could have very easily suffered the many dangerous side effects.

4

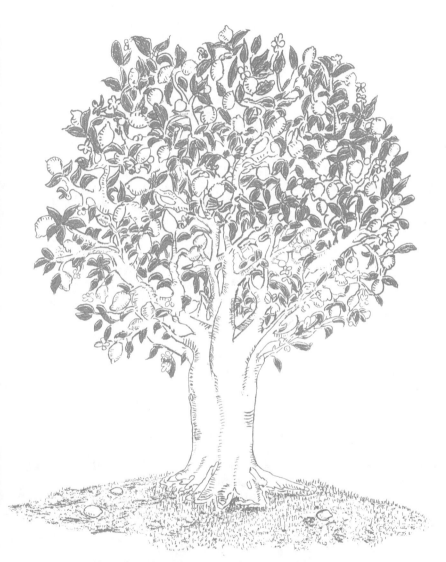

LEMONS AND LIMES
our family tree of life

The Origin of the Lemonade Diet

The lemonade diet, about to be described, has successfully and consistently demonstrated its eliminative and building ability. It may be used with complete safety for every known type of disease.

Lemons and limes are the richest source of minerals and vitamins of any food or foods known to man, and they are available the year round. Thus the diet may be used successfully any month of the year and virtually any place on earth. Its universal appeal and availability make it pleasant and easy to use.

The lemonade diet first proved itself in the healing of stomach ulcers over forty years ago. Permission was given by Bob Norman to share this incident of my first experience with the diet.

One day, shortly prior to my first meeting with Bob, I was inspired to write this diet in complete form as a means to give relief and to heal stomach ulcers in ten days. I rapidly wrote it down in detail and waited for a test case — which always seemed to come when it was needed.

Bob Norman had suffered with his ulcer for nearly three years. During this time he had tried everything then known to get help, but nothing in the way of medicine or treatment gave anything but momentary relief. He had to eat something every two hours or he was in extreme pain. For the preceding three months he had been living on little other than goats milk. His doctor wanted to operate but he refused to have it done. He figured anything would be better than that. He told me I was the last person he would go to. If I couldn't help him, he would just go home and die, as life was hardly worth living in this condition.

An explanation of the cause of an ulcer is necessary at this point. There is a sodium coating covering the entire inside wall of the stomach which, if it remains intact, will prevent the digestive juices from digesting the stomach itself. However, when any form of flesh food enters the stomach, the meat attracts the sodium in the same way as the walls of the stomach. Some of the sodium is drawn from the walls and gathers around the meat, thus preventing the digestion of the meat in the stomach and at the same time depleting the sodium on the walls of the stomach.

As one continues to eat meat and a deficiency of sodium in the diet occurs, the sodium lining is not being replaced on the walls of the stomach. The digestive juices then start digesting the stomach, producing what we call an ulcer. When this occurs, all orthodox methods to heal the ulcer fail completely.

Sometimes the meat can remain in the stomach for two or more hours and begin to ferment and spoil. To be broken down and digested it must pass on into the small intestine. All forms of meat take longer to digest than do fruit and vegetables. Chicken and other fowl take the longest of all. Just because meat is already a form of flesh, it does not follow that it is readily usable by our bodies. In fact, just the reverse is true.

When one considers that flesh foods of all kinds are extremely toxic, it becomes apparent that they are an extremely undesireable form of nourishment. In the eating of meat, one must take into account all of our eliminative organs. They are made primarily to take care of **our own wastes.** When we add animal flesh, containing the wastes of its cells (or drugs and other unusable materials), extra work is required of these organs and various forms of trouble will eventually develop.

Remember that all solid food must be broken down into a liquid form to be carried by the blood before it can nourish the body. Flesh foods of all kinds (including fish) take much longer to reach this state and are less useful to the body than fruit, vegetables, and seeds.

Back to our story. After all of Bob's explanation, I asked him if he would like to have his ulcer healed in ten days. He answered "Yes" so I handed him the paper with the diet on it. He read it over carefully and handed it back with the explanation that he could never do that as all expert advice for three years had told him to never use citrus, and this was nothing but lemonade.

Since orthodox methods had failed completely to heal his ulcer, I reasoned that their advice could be wrong. And since the lemonade diet was **contrary** to the accepted practices (which had failed), logic told me that it might do the healing. I knew it could do no harm and was confident only good could come from it.

I explained to Bob that if all of this expert advice was correct, his ulcer would have been healed three years ago! It was just possible that the very thing he was told not to use might be the one thing he needed. He thought it over and decided, "All right, I'll try it . . . even if it kills me!" He was assured that this would not happen.

After five days of the diet Bob called me. Even though he had no pain from the beginning, he was afraid that suddenly all the old pain would return and he would be miserable again. Formerly he had to eat something every two hours or he would be in pain, and the previous day he had gone eight hours without food or drink — with no pain, yet he was still apprehensive. I assured him that since he had no pain for five days, he would be all right and to continue for the full ten days.

On the eleventh day he was examined by his doctor and the ulcer had been completely healed. Needless to say, his doctor was most amazed because he had given Bob a complete examination, including X-ray, prior to the diet and had recommended an immediate operation because he would not have long to live otherwise.

Many more cases of ulcers followed with the same consistant results in only ten days with no failures.

But something else happened that I was not looking for – in every case the client had other disorders – such as – sinus, asthma, hay fever, bronchial disorders, colds, flu, arthritis and other allergies which completely cleared up or greatly improved in the ten day period.

Much to my pleasant surprise – I had discovered a principal that had the natural ability to heal all disorders without any complications or side effects. Suddenly the use of any forms of drugs or chemicals were no longer required or desired for any disease since they have never accomplished the desired healing. They have only treated the diseases but never healed. ALL FORMS OF MEDICATION HAVE THEIR DANGEROUS SIDE EFFECTS SINCE MEDICATION DOES NO WORK IN HARMONY WITH NATURE AND THE NATURAL NEEDS OF THE BODY IN ITS ORIGINAL MAKEUP.

Next I needed to spend much time in complete research as to why the lemonade was the finest in correcting all diseases.

Little by little the answers came as thousands of sufferers continued to get well and free of their afflictions. The lemonade contained all the vitamins and minerals – with no exceptions – for an indefinite length of time. Tests were made before and after the diet and in every case where there were shortages of any kind – to begin with – there were no deficiencies at the end of the diet at any time and if there were no shortages in the beginning – which was rare – there were still no shortages at the end. This was amazing – a miracle – that anything so simple could supply all the needs of the body so easily with no complications of formulas of other foods.

The Master Cleanser
By Herman Schneider

MISSING A MEAL WON'T HURT!

Since the days of Jesus Christ, who fasted for 40 days, men and women have abstained from food for many reasons; for health, for political ends, and for spiritual enlightment.

However, the average person, not familiar with fasting, believes he will certainly die if he misses a meal. When you hear of a person dying after lost in the woods or at sea for two or three days, it was not lack of food that caused his death, but it was panic and fear that killed him. Most people in fairly good health can go for many days without food but the body must have water, although there is a fast called "the dry fast" which employs dry bread but no liquid. However, this type of fast cannot be endured for too long a period.

There is general disagreement in the health field on the best way to detoxify the body. The Hygienists, who are mostly followers of Dr. Herbert Shelton, the very capable exponent of fasting, using only distilled water, and enemas are taboo. Dr. Shelton and other Hygienist doctors have fasted thousands of people, many regaining their health, as a result of the fast. Of course, after the fast, it was necessary for them to follow a healthful way of life. The Hygienists are strict vegetarians with the emphasis on raw foods and proper combinations.

Dr. Walker and Dr. Airola advocate fruit and vegetable juice if fasting is needed. In Europe naturopaths use the vegetable broth and vegetable juice fast rather than the water fast. The above doctors also employ colonics and enemas, these being vital for the success of the program. The purpose, in their opinion, is to rid the body of the toxins loosened by the cleanse.

Thirteen years ago I had extremely high blood pressure. I didn't feel too well so I went to the doctor. He gulped as he said to me, "your blood pressure of 200 over 120."

He told me that he would start me on medication but I did not think that drugs were the answer for me so I asked him, "How long do I have to stay on drugs?" He replied, "Your hypertension will get progressively worse so you will have to stay on the medicine forever." He continued, "in thirty years of practice I have only had two patients able to discontinue the medicine."

I was not pleased with his answer so I said, "You are looking at your third patient who will get off the medicine."

He looked at me and shrugged his shoulders as if to say, "He is insane." He said, "I have hundreds of patients on medications for high blood pressure, and you are the only one who makes a fuss."

I took one drug for a week but it made me dizzy so he changed the medicine. he gave me one drug for high blood pressure and another for nerves, which slowed me down; then another drug to pep me up from the drug that was slowing me down.

CHANGED PROGRAM

I decided this program was not for me so I headed for Dr. Shelton's in San Antonio, Texas, they took all my drugs and threw them away and put me to bed to start my fast. I never dreamt I would go without food so long but my fast lasted for 21 days on just distilled water.

It is during the fast that conditions a person may have but is not yet aware of, show up, as the body begins throwing off the poisons. The man fasting in the next room passed gallstones on his 24th day. He never knew he had gallstones before his fast. He really suffered until he passed his stones. After long years of study in natural healing and herbology I now know he could have gotten rid of the gallstones in a much more pleasant way, using apple juice, olive oil and lemon juice.

I, myself, had mild reactions outside of extreme weakness. My biggest problem was painful cramps caused by gas in the intestines. I also had some bleeding as the bowel tried to empty itself with no bulk ingested to help it move.

My fasting problems would have been much less had they given me an enema, but the Hygienists do not believe in enemas, laxitives or herbs. They say nature must take its course.

The faster is kept in bed most of the time, using one's energy to detoxify.

On the 21 days of fasting I lost 21 pounds, which I gradually gained back during the rebuilding process, which should equal the fasting time. So I had to stay off of my job for 42 days.

The fast was not pleasant, although you lose your desire for food after the third day. But the results were very pleasant and made it worthwhile; my blood pressure was now 120 over 80 which is perfect.

Since this fast, thirteen years ago, I have fasted many times on vegetable juices and used colonics as advocated by Dr. Walker. The fasts were of short duration, lasting from two to five days.

About a year ago I went to a chiropractor for an adjustment. We talked for a while and he told me he was on a lemon juice cleanse, so I asked for details. He sold me a book called the "Master Cleanser" by Stanley Burroughs, a natural healer for some forty or more years.

The cleanse starts with a herbal laxative tea both morning and evening. If this is not sufficient to clean out the intestinal tract he advises a salt water wash. These steps are necessary to remove the toxins, loosened by the lemon juice cleanse.

I was then to drink between six and twelve glasses of lemonade, which consisted of lemon and maple syrup in proper proportions, with a small amount of cayenne added to wash out the mucous loosened by the cleanse.

Mr. Burrough's book, "The Master Cleanser" describes the entire program, including directions for diabetics to get off insulin. I, myself, believe that diabetics should be under the care of their doctors, if they choose to follow the Burroughs program. For diabetics, he does not advocate that they use maple syrup in the beginning but to use black-strap molasses. Lemon juice, maple syrup and blackstrap molasses are very high in all minerals and vitamins.

I stayed on the "Master Cleanse" for 12 days, during which I exercised, jogged, worked, and felt stronger each day, as the cleanse proceeded. I gradually tapered off the cleanse, with juices and broth, for three more days. During the entire time I was never hungry.

The most important part of the cleanse or any fast is knowing how to come off of the fast, allowing the body to gradually adjust itself to handling solid food again. Improper procedures can cause illness and even death.

Since my weight was stabilized when I started the cleanse, I only lost about four pounds in twelve days. People who are overweight will lose much more.

Mr. Burroughs' program calls for a vegetarian diet so this part of the program was easy for me to accept because I have been a vegetarian for years, using mostly raw foods.

I go on this cleanse two or three times a year. I just read in Linda Clark's book that she has used this cleanse for years.

Mr. Burroughs says that it is perfectly safe to stay on the "Master Cleanser" even up to 40 days, as the lemon, maple syrup or blackstrap molasses and cayenne pepper act as both a cleanser, and a body builder.

From my viewpoint the Burroughs cleanse gave me the best results, allowing me to be active and energetic through the entire period.

I haven't been back to the medical doctors but my blood pressure is still normal after all these years.

NOTE

THE FOLLOWING DIET IS GIVEN SOLELY AS A SUGGESTION; ANYONE WHO FOLLOWS IT DOES SO VOLUNTARILY. SINCE EACH PER-SON, NATURALLY, REACTS DIFFERENTLY, EACH INDIVIDUAL MUST USE HIS OWN JUDGEMENT AS TO ITS USE.

The Master Cleanser
or
The Lemonade Diet

Purpose

To dissolve and eliminate toxins and congestion that have formed in any part of the body.
To cleanse the kidneys and the digestive system.
To purify the glands and cells throughout the entire body.
To eliminate all unusable waste and hardened material in the joints and muscles.
To relieve pressure and irritation in the nerves, arteries, and blood vessels.
To build a healthy blood stream.
To keep youth and elasticity regardless of our years.

When to Use It

When sickness has developed — for all acute and chronic conditions.
When the digestive system needs a rest and a cleansing.
When overweight has become a problem.
When better assimilation and building of body tissue is needed.

And How Often?

Follow the diet for a minimum of 10 days or more — up to 40 days and beyond may be safely followed for extremely serious cases. The diet has all the nutrition needed during this time. Three to four times a year will do wonders for keeping the body in a normal healthy condition. The diet may be undertaken more frequently for serious conditions.

How to Make It

2 Tbsp lemon or lime juice (approx. ½ lemon)
2 Tbsp genuine maple syrup (not maple flavored sugar syrup)
1/10 Tsp cayenne pepper (red pepper) or to taste
Water, medium hot (spring or purified water)

Combine the juice, maple syrup, and cayenne pepper in a 10 oz. glass and fill with medium hot water. (Cold water may be used if preferred.)

Use fresh lemons or limes only, never canned lemon or lime juice nor frozen lemonade or frozen juice. Use organic lemons when possible.

The maple syrup is a balanced form of positive and negative sugar and must be used, not some "substitute". There are three grades of

12

maple syrup. Grade A is the first run — mild in taste, sweet and with less minerals than the other grades. It is more expensive and less desirable but it may be used. Grade B is the second run with more minerals plus more maple taste. It is more suitable for the diet and is less expensive. Grade C is the third run with even more minerals and still stronger taste of maple and slightly less pleasant for most people, although acceptable in the diet. It is lower in price. As Grade C is less expensive it can be used as an excellent sweetening agent in preparing foods. The strong maple flavor blends very well.

The maple syrup has a large variety of minerals and vitamins. Naturally the mineral and vitamin content will vary according to the area where the trees grow and the mineral content in the soil. These are the minerals found in average samples of syrup from Vermont: Sodium; Potassium; Calcium; Magnesium; Manganese; Iron; Copper; Phosphorus; Sulphur; Chlorine and Silicon. Vitamin A, B1, B2, B6, C, Nicotinic acid and Pantothenic acid are also present in the syrup. Information on the need and effect of these properties will be found in the Biochemistry in the back of the book.

Some uninformed operators of the sugaring of the maple syrup do use formaldehyde pellets, run through polyethylene tubing but there are many more that don't. Search out and demand the kind not using formaldehyde.

Dozens of letters weekly, from around the world highly praise the many superior benefits of the lemonade diet. Thus, we must conclude that since it does so much for so many it is truly The Master Cleanser. The following is a quote from one of the letters: "I tried the lemonade diet with exceptionally beneficial results. I would like to order at least six at whatever your wholesale price would be — I know I will need many more as I do push the books. I believe they are the best in their field."

An ideal formula involves freshly extracted juice from the sugar cane (readily available in India, but not generally in the United States at the present time):

10 oz. fresh sugar cane juice (medium hot or cold)

2 tbsp. fresh lime or lemon juice

1/10 tsp cayenne (red pepper) or to taste

Another possible but lesser replacement could be pure sorghum. (Do not use for Diabetes). It does not produce equal or close to the benefits of maple syrup.

Special Instructions for the Diabetic

DIABETES is the result of a deficiency diet consisting in part of white sugar and white flour. The lemonade with molasses is an ideal way to correct this deficiency. FOLLOW THE DIRECTIONS CAREFULLY FOR BEST RESULTS. The molasses supplies the necessary elements for the pancreas to produce insulin. As the necessary elements are supplied to the pancreas, the amount of insulin taken may also be gradually reduced -- as an example.

ON THE FIRST DAY use a scant tablespoon of molasses to each glass of lemonade and reduce insulin by about 10 units. Daily from then on reduce the insulin as you increase the molasses to 2 full tablespoons per glass. When this proportion has been reached the insulin can normally be eliminated; then replace the molasses with 2 tablespoons of maple syrup in each glass. Make regular checks of the sugar level in the urine and blood to satisfy yourself and eliminate any possible fear. Vita Flex and color therapy may be used to advantage to stimulate the liver, pancreas, and spleen and thus insure proper use of the minerals supplied. Many people have found they no longer have need for insulin. They must be sure to follow every detail of the recommended diet as explained in the following pages.

What About the Use of Honey?

Honey must not be used at any time internally. It is manufactured from the nectar picked up from the flowers by the bees — good enough in itself, perhaps — then predigested, vomited and stored for their own future use with a preservative added. It is deficient in calcium and has many detrimental effects for the human being.

According to one authority, honey is "a magical and mystical word in Healthfoodland. It is one of the most overpromoted, overpriced product being sold to gullible health foodists. The great value attributed to honey is delusive . . . honey is only a little less empty and more dangerous than sugar."

Just as with alcohol, honey, being predigested, enters the blood directly, raising the sugar content very rapidly above normal. To correct this, the pancreas must produce insulin immediately or possible death can occur. More insulin than necessary is likely to be produced, and the blood sugar level then drops below normal. This can produce blackout spells and even death if it goes too low. When blood sugar is below normal, a person will feel depressed. The regular use of honey can create constant imbalances which in turn will adversely affect the normal function of the liver, pancreas and spleen. Hypoglycemia and hyperglycemia are the results of the use of unbalanced sugars. The balanced sugar in maple syrup and sugar cane juice causes no dangerous side effects. All natural fruits and vegetables have balanced sugars in them. Artificial, synthetic, and refined sugars have no place in a natural diet.

Is the Lemonade Diet Also a Reducing Diet?

As a reducing diet it is superior in every way to any other system because it dissolves and eliminates all types of fatty tissue. Fat melts away at the rate of about two pounds a day for most persons — and without any harmful side effects.

All mucus diseases such as colds, flu, asthma, hay fever, sinus and bronchial troubles are rapidly dissolved and eliminated from the body, leaving the user free from the varied allergies which cause difficult breathing and clogging of the sinus cavities. Allergies exist as a result of an accumulation of these toxins and they vanish as we cleanse our body. People who are over-weight often experience these difficulties, and the more they continue to eat the toxic fat-producing foods which cause their obesity, the more their other ailments multiply.

Mucus disorders are brought about by the eating or drinking of mucus-forming foods. In other words, if you have these diseases, **you ate them!** As we stop feeding our family mucus-forming foods, we can eliminate their mucus and allergy diseases for the rest of their lives.

The types of disease which are a result of calcium deposits in the joints, muscles, cells and glands are readily dissolved and removed from the body. Cholesterol deposits in the arteries and veins also respond to the magic cleansing power of the lemonade diet.

All skin disorders also disappear as the rest of the body is cleansed. Boils, abscesses, carbuncles, and pimples all come under this category. These conditions are, again, Nature's effort to eliminate poisons quickly from the body.

All types of infections are the result of these vast accumulations of poisons being dissolved and burned or oxidized to produce further cleansing of the body. Therefore, rapid elimination of the toxins relieves the need for infectious fevers of all kinds. Infections are not "caught," they are created by Nature to assist in burning our surplus wastes.

Yes, the lemonade diet is a reducing diet, **but much more.** Just as many other disorders also cleared up at the same time when it was used to heal ulcers, when it is used as a reducing diet other ailments are also corrected in the process.

People build strong, healthy bodies from the correct foods or they build diseased bodies from incorrect foods. When disease does become necessary, the lemonade diet will prove its superior cleansing and building ability.

Blend a part of the lemon skin and pulp with the lemonade in a blender for further cleansing and laxative effect. (Note: commercially procured lemons may have had their skins dyed with yellow coloring and may have been subjected to poisonous insect sprays — be sure to peel off the outer skin if you cannot get uncolored, organically grown lemons.) The properties in the lemon skin also act as a hemostatic to prevent excess bleeding and to prevent clotting internally should there be any such prevailing condition. (Don't worry — normal conditions will continue during the menstrual periods.)

Adding the cayenne pepper is necessary as it breaks up mucus and increases warmth by building the blood for an additional lift. It also adds many of the B and C vitamins.

Mint tea may be used occasionally during this diet as a pleasant change and to assist further in the cleansing. Its chlorophyll helps as a purifier, neutralizing many mouth and body odors that are released during the cleansing period.

How Much Does One Drink?

Take from six to twelve glasses of the lemonade daily during the waking period. As you get hungry just have another glass of lemonade. NO OTHER FOOD SHOULD BE TAKEN DURING THE FULL PERIOD OF THE DIET. As this is a complete balance of minerals and vitamins, one does not suffer the pangs of hunger. Do not use vitamin pills.

All solid food is turned into a liquid state before it can be carried by the blood to the cells of the body. The lemonade is already a food in liquid form.

For those who are overweight, less maple syrup may be taken. For those underweight, more maple syrup may be taken. For those who are underweight and worried about losing more weight, REMEMBER, the only things you can possibly lose are mucus, waste, and disease. Healthy tissue will not be eliminated. Many people who need to gain weight actually do so near the end of the diet period.

Never vary the amount of lemon juice per glass. About six glasses of lemonade a day is enough for those wishing to reduce. Extra water may be taken as desired.

Helping the Cleansing Along

As this is a cleansing diet, the more you can assist Nature to eliminate poisons, the better. **If your system feels upset, it is because you are not having sufficient elimination.** Avoid this possibility by following the directions completely. Above all, be sure you have two, three, or more movements a day. This may seem unnecessary not eating solid food, but it is Nature's way of eliminating the waste it has loosened from the various cells and organs in the body. They must leave the body some way. It would be just the same as sweeping the floor around and around and never removing the dirt from the house if the wastes were not passed out. The better the elimination, the more rapid will be the results.

A LAXATIVE HERB TEA is found to be the best helper for most persons. It is a good practice to take a good laxative herb tea right from the beginning — the last thing at night and first thing in the morning. There are several good laxative teas. They are best taken in a liquid form. Buy them in your health food store.

Another Cleansing Aid: Internal Salt Water Bathing

As it is necessary to bathe the outside of our bodies, so it is with the inside. Do not take enemas or colonics at any time during the cleansing diet or afterwards. They are unnecessary and can be extremely harmful.

There is a much superior method of cleansing the colonic tract without the harmful effects of customary colonics and enemas. This method will cleanse the entire digestive tract while the colonics and enemas will only reach the colon or a small part of it. Colonics can be expensive while our salt water method is not.

DIRECTIONS: Prepare a full quart of luke-warm water and add two level (rounded for the Canadian quart) teaspoons of uniodized sea salt. Do not use ordinary iodized salt as it will not work properly. Drink the entire quart of salt and water first thing in the morning. This must be taken on an empty stomach. The salt and water will not separate but will stay intact and quickly and thoroughly wash the entire tract in about one hour. Several eliminations will likely occur. The salt water has the same specific gravity as the blood, hence the kidneys cannot pick up the water and the blood cannot pick up the salt. This may be taken as often as needed for proper washing of the entire digestive system.

If the salt water does not work the first time, try adding a little more or a little less salt until the proper balance is found; or possibly take extra water with or without salt. This often increases the activity. Remember, it can do no harm at any time. The colon needs a good washing, but do it the natural way — the salt water way.

It is quite advisable to take the herb laxative tea at night to loosen, then the salt water each morning to wash it out. If for some reason the salt water cannot be taken in the morning, then the herb laxative tea must be taken night and morning.

Should I Take "Supplements"?

Some people want to take vitamin pills or food supplements while on the diet. This frequently fails to produce the desired result. There are many reasons. As the lymphatic glands become clogged, they are no longer able to assimilate and digest even the best of foods. As we cleanse our bodies and free our cells and glands of toxins that clog and paralyze our assimilation, we free our various organs and processes to do their proper jobs. Note below. All the necessary vitamins and minerals are in the lemonade, and therefore we do not need an additional supply in most cases.

Vitamin pills and supplements do not grow on trees as such but rather come to us in fruits, berries, vegetables and plants. Man will never take a group of natural or synthetic foods; process and combine them in a variety of products, and come up with anything equal or better than the original. They have lost much of their basic life and energy by combining them according to a man made concept. Many dangerous side effects can occur because of improper and unequal balances present. Stay with the natural laws of balance. First one must decide if God is right or if man is right. If God is right then man and his ideas of processing — tearing apart and rearranging — are likely to be wrong.

Later, as we consume a more complete variety of foods, we find our sources of vitamins and minerals complete and in forms that are easily assimilated — it should not be necessary to return to these supplements even if one is accustomed to taking them. The sources of good food are steadily being enlarged as people become more educated concerning them. Search these sources and rely on them for your total nutritional needs.

The lemon is a loosening and cleansing agent with many important building factors. The ability of the elements in the lemon and the maple syrup working together creates these desired results.

Its 49% potassium strengthens and energizes the heart, stimulates and builds the kidneys and adrenal glands.

Its oxygen builds vitality.

Its carbon acts as a motor stimulant.

Its hydrogen activates the sensory nervous system.

Its calcium strengthens and builds the lungs.

Its phosphorus knits the bones, stimulates and builds the brain for clearer thinking.

Its sodium encourages tissue building.

Its magnesium acts as a blood alkalizer.

Its iron builds the red corpuscles to rapidly correct the most common forms of anemia.

Its chlorine cleanses the blood plasma.

Its silicon aids the thyroid for deeper breathing.

The natural iron, copper, calcium, carbon, and hydrogen found in the sweetening supplies more building and cleansing material. It truly is a perfect combination for cleansing, eliminating, healing, and building. Hence, supplements are not needed during the diet and may actually interfere with its cleansing action.

Will It Make Me Feel Bad or Weak?

In the cleansing process, some people experience a tremendous stirring up and may even feel worse for several days. It is not the lemonade that causes the trouble, but what the lemonade stirs up in the system that causes our dizziness and other disturbances. Vomiting may occur under certain conditions; increased pain may be felt in the various joints of the body; dizziness may develop on certain days. If weakness develops at any time, it is the result of poisons circulating through the blood stream rather than a lack of food or vitamins. This diet gives a person all the vitamins, food, and energy necessary for the full ten days or longer in a liquid form. Rest and take it a little easier if you have to — although most people can go on about their regular business without difficulty. Keep right on with the diet; don't give up or "cheat" by eating a little food or you may destroy the benefits.

Even though the lemon is an acid fruit, it becomes alkaline as it is digested and assimilated. It is, in fact, our best aid toward proper alkaline balance. There is no danger of "too much acid."

Alcoholics, smokers, and other drug addicts will receive untold benefits from this diet. The chemical changes and the cleansing have a way of removing the craving and the many probable deficiencies. Thus the desire for the unnatural types of stimulants and depressants disappears. The usual cravings experienced and suffered in breaking away from drugs, alcohol, and tobacco no longer present themselves during and after this diet.

It is truly a wonderful feeling to be free from slavery to these many habit-forming and devitalizing elements of modern living. Coffee, tea, and various cola drinks, as habit-forming beverages, also lose their appeal through the marvels of the lemonade diet.

How to Break the Lemonade Diet

Coming off the lemonade diet properly is highly important — please follow the directions very carefully. After living in a semi-tropical and tropical climate for many years, I find that people have increasingly turned to a raw fruit, nut, and vegetable diet. Following is the schedule for people who normally follow such a natural vegetarian diet:

FIRST and SECOND DAY AFTER DIET:
Several 8 oz. glasses of fresh orange juice as desired during the day.

The orange juice prepares the digestive system to properly digest and assimilate regular food. Drink it slowly. If there has been any digestive difficulty prior to or during the change over, extra water may be taken with the orange juice.

THIRD DAY:
Orange juice in the morning. Raw fruit for lunch. Fruit or raw vegetable salad at night. You are now ready to eat normally.

For those who have characteristically lived the unnatural way of meat, milk, refined and devitalized food, it may be best to change over as follows, gradually adopting the raw fruit, nut, and vegetable diet:

FIRST DAY:
Several 8 oz. glasses of fresh orange juice as desired during the day. Drink it slowly.

SECOND DAY:
Drink several 8 oz. glasses of orange juice during the day — with extra water, if needed. Some time during the afternoon prepare a vegetable soup (no canned soup) as follows:

Recipe for Vegetable Soup

Use several kinds of vegetables, perhaps one or two kinds of legumes, potatoes, celery, carrots, green vegetable tops, onion, etc. Dehydrated vegetables or vegetable soup powders may be added for extra flavor. Okra or okra powder, chili, curry, cayenne (red) pepper, tomatoes, green peppers, and zucchini squash may be included to good advantage. Brown rice may be used, but no meat or meat stock. Other spices may be added (delicately) for flavor. Use salt delicately as a limited amount of salt is necessary. Learn to enjoy the natural flavor of the vegetables. The less cooking the better. Read the special article on salt in the September 1977 issue of National Geographic magazine.

Have this soup for the evening meal using the broth mostly, although some of the vegetables may be eaten. Rye wafers may be eaten sparingly with the soup, but no bread or crackers.

THIRD DAY:
Drink orange juice in the morning. At noon have some more soup; enough may be made the night before and put in the refrigerator. For the evening meal eat whatever is desired in the form of vegetables, salads, or fruit. No meat, fish, or eggs; no bread, pastries, tea, coffee,

or milk. Milk is highly mucus-forming and tends to develop toxins throughout the body.

(Milk, being a predigested food, has been known to cause various complications in the stomach and colon, such as cramps and convulsions. The calcium in milk is difficult to assimilate and may cause toxins in the form of rheumatic fever, arthritis, neuritis, and bursitis. The resulting lack of proper digestion and assimilation of the calcium allows it to go into the blood stream in a free form and it is deposited in the tissues, cells, and joints where it can cause intense pain and suffering.)

FOURTH DAY:
Normal eating may be resumed, but best health will be retained if the morning meal consists of our type of lemonade or fruit juice; and, of course, if a strictly fruit, vegetable, seed and berry diet is followed. If, after eating is resumed, distress or gas occurs, it is suggested that the lemonade diet be continued for several more days until the system is ready for food.

Recap of the steps to be taken in the diet. Be careful to read the entire instructions so that the diet will be of the best benefit to you.

First prepare yourself mentally to follow in detail the entire directions and continue as long as is needed to make the necessary changes. One of the best signals of the completed diet is when the formerly coated and fuzzy tongue is clear pink and clean looking. During the diet it becomes very badly coated.

The Night Before starting the diet take the laxative tea.

In the morning take the salt water (or) laxative tea (see page 15 for details). This should be done each night and morning during the diet — rare exception — if diarrhea develops. When diarrhea is ended then continue above directions.

Now the lemonade formula (see page 10 for details or page 13 if diabetic).

Breaking the diet. Be absolutely sure you follow the directions very carefully to prepare your body for normal eating (our way). Do not over eat or eat too soon. Serious problems (nausea) can occur if detailed directions are not followed.

How Do I Get My Protein?

Often the question is asked about the need for amino acids, and animal protein foods. The need is highly exaggerated as only 16% of our body is protein. The answer to the question is very simple. We first need to understand that pure protein is primarily nitrogen, with oxygen, hydrogen and some carbon. We all know we get a large share of our oxygen and hydrogen needs from the air along with some carbon. There is four times the amount of nitrogen in the same air as there is oxygen, hydrogen and carbon combined. Since we are able to utilize and assimilate a large amount of our needs of these elements into our bodies we are able to assimilate and build the nitrogen also into our bodies as protein. This is done by natural bacteria action which is capable of converting it to our use.

From the combination of the best of foods and clean air we are able to create our own amino acids, just as well as the animals do. We never try to feed amino acids to the animals. Thus we are able to eliminate the need for toxic dead animal flesh and have no further need to worry about our constant source of protein. Eat only the best variety of fruits, berries, nuts, vegetables, seeds and sprouted seeds for a further complete source of protein.

People who smoke cannot pick up the nitrogen from the air so easily, but will still get enough from proper food without the use of animal flesh. For your well being, however, elimination of smoking is a must.

Many people believe that eating meat gives them strength. If this is so, then why are the strongest animals in the world vegetarians? Did you ever stop to think that the animals you do eat are vegetarian? Where did they get their strength? All the meat-eating animals find it necessary to sleep 16 to 18 hours daily because of excess toxins. The meat eating animals live a very short life. God has supplied such a bountiful supply of fresh, wholesome food that there is never a need to kill an animal for its more toxic flesh in our modern civilization.

Feeding Your Baby

All babies should be nursed by the mother if at all possible. There is no real substitute. Cows and goats milk is for their babies and is not suitable for the human baby. It creates mucus and other problems just the same as in adults, including colds and infectious diseases.

Correct food, reflex stimulation, and color therapy will assure the mother all the milk she needs for her baby. Where mother's milk is not available the best replacement is coconut milk — see recipe on page 32. With this, give the baby about 8 ounces of lemonade in between regular feedings. To the regular formula for lemonade add about double the amount of water until the infant is about six months old and then gradually change to regular strength. A nursing baby should begin to be weaned in nine months and be eating regular foods after that.

Commercially prepared baby foods and baby formulas are unfit for the balanced need of a healthy baby. Recent articles and TV reports indicate these foods are very undesirable **always.** Prepare fresh food from fruit, vegetables, berries, and seeds. The baby has no need for any of the animal or fish products. Use pure maple syrup instead of sugar or honey when sweetening is needed. Your baby deserves only the very best of live fresh foods. Caring for a healthy baby is a great pleasure with fewer problems when this pattern is followed. At the same time it develops good lifelong habits of sound nutrition.

Is Water Fasting a Good Thing?

The subject of water fasting often presents itself. I am very much opposed to several days or weeks of water fasting. It is too dangerous and is unnecessary to achieve the desired results of internal cleansing.

Many people are already deficient as well as toxic. The longer they do without food, the greater becomes the deficiency. The lemonade diet can more than match all the possible good obtained from fasting and at the same time will rebuild any possible deficiency.

Ordinarily with fasting it is necessary to take it easy by resting or staying in bed. On the contrary, with the lemonade diet there is no need to become a useless member of society — you may live an active, normal life. Many workers at hard labor have found they are able to do more and harder work while on the lemonade diet than on their normal diet.

After one has attained a clean, healthy body, and then desires to fast for purely spiritual reasons, thirty or even forty days can cause no harm. First we must build our physical bodies to their highest condition.

Your friends and acquaintances may find this lemonade diet to be the answer to their aches, pains, or other troubles. Even if there appears to be nothing wrong, sometimes those who are "never sick" will feel even better. Let your friends receive this benefit too.

A Gift of Life to Sheila

Around the year of 1958 we gave a class in Hemet, California. A Mr. & Mrs. C. were in this class. During the next few years they accomplished many wonderful things in healing. One of their most outstanding cases would stand out as truly a miracle in any field or system of healing.

Some time in 1963 Mr. C. took on the responsibility of raising and caring for his great niece at the age of 3½ weeks. She was diagnosed by the medical doctor as hopeless and beyond any form of help to his knowledge. He expected her to die within a few days. There was nothing medicine had to offer as a life saver. He told the parents "Take her home and enjoy her for a few days as she has not long to live."

The couple accepting the responsibility, proceeded to feed and care for her with natural methods. The feeding consisted of fresh lemonade, orange juice and carrot juice for about three years. Gradually she was fed other natural raw foods — no animal milk or processed foods. Treatments consisted of the color therapy and Vita-Flex as a part of the healing and building process.

I had the special privilege of seeing this girl at the age of 14 years. The beauty and the poise of the girl was most outstanding. She is now an accomplished organist, pianist, opera singer and artist in painting.

She was raised without any form of animal products and has never had any form of medication, operation or shots. Also during these 14 years she has had none of the diseases that other children have when raised by the orthodox methods.

Sheila came to me at our first meeting and stated rather emotionally, "Mr. Burroughs, you have no idea how much we appreciate you — because without you and your system I could not have lived."

At that moment I thought to myself how wonderful that through my strong and constant desire I had created a system that had saved her life and could save the life of many other hopeless cases like hers if only the entire world knew about it.

Suddenly all of the countless years of frustrations I had encountered in producing this work seemed to disappear and this made everything all worth while. The thrill of knowing and using this knowledge to bring life more abundant to a suffering world knows no bounds.

This case, like many other cases prove that, when we work knowingly with all the natural laws, diseases, as we know them, no longer exist. This work must go on and be available to everyone no matter who or where they are.

A New Treatment for an Old Ailment: DROPSY (EDEMA)

Dropsy is one of the most difficult and least understood of the many expressions of toxemia. It consists of an accumulation of fluid in the body tissues. Varied attempts to correct this condition have met with little or no success. The main treatments can give only temporary relief and the final result, as these treatments fail to produce any change, is death from internal drowning.

To achieve fast relief and lasting correction, one must completely understand the causes. Then our unusual and simple approach to an ancient disease will achieve quick and lasting results.

As with so many other diseases, dropsy represents a vast accumulation of toxic wastes. These toxins accumulate because our eliminative organs are unable to take care of them as fast as they enter or are formed in the body. As accumulations steadily increase, they first appear to us in liquid form. If they are not eliminated from our body, they are automatically and gradually dehydrated or crystallized. They are then deposited in any and all of the available spaces throughout our cells, glands, and organs. This continues until a saturation point is reached and then Nature reverses the action and slowly dissolves the crystallized and dehydrated material. This change is the body's final effort to save the life from being snuffed out from complete stoppage of all glands and organs. Only in a liquid or semi-liquid form can we eliminate our toxins. Usually, by this time our eliminative organs are overworked and clogged, our heart, liver, and kidneys suffering the most, so they cannot carry off the liquid toxins. The body then steadily increases in size until it can no longer sustain life.

The correction for this otherwise fatal condition is simple, fast, and effective. Just follow directions and the results will be most satisfactory.

Now, the treatment. Start the patient off on the lemonade diet. This begins the internal cleansing process.

Next, secure one hundred (100) pounds of coarse rock salt (which may be purchased at a feed store). Cover the bottom of the bath tub with about two inches of salt. Unclothe the patient and wrap the person in a wet sheet. Then lay the patient on the salt and add salt to about two inches above their body so that the entire body is surrounded with the salt. The room should be 80° or slightly higher so the patient does not get chilled. (The tub may be warmed first with hot water before adding the salt. Let ALL the water out first before adding the salt.)

Leave the patient in the salt for approximately one hour. Be sure you have given them several glasses of hot lemonade with cayenne pepper in advance.

Remove the patient from the salt and wrap them in a woolen blanket to keep them warm. Extra heat may be used if necessary. Repeat this treatment every other day or daily, if not too weak from the rapid changes.

This may be repeated until all the swelling has gone down or the toxins are removed. The first application may not produce notable results. but from then on a rapid change should be observed.

Be sure to keep the dropsy victim on the lemonade diet until a big change has taken place, even if it continues for ten, twenty, or thirty days. Color and Vita-Flex may be used also and will provide tremendously increased action and elimination.

IMPORTANT NOTE: The salt may be used over and over on the same patient, but not on any other. Each person must have their own salt.

Bathing one or two times a day, especially during this diet, is especially necessary. We eliminate wastes through the breathing, the skin, the kidneys, the colon and from the sinus through the nose. The most wastes are eliminated by breathing; next in order are the skin, the colon, the kidneys, and depending on the individual, from the sinus. Often we eliminate large quantities of wastes in the form of mucus as we develop colds or flu. One can see how important becomes our elimination by the skin. Even when in good condition, it is important to bathe once or twice daily to remove these wastes from the surface of the skin, thus allowing it to breathe properly. These baths will help to eliminate obnoxious odors while we cleanse our body. Frequent steam baths will also help.

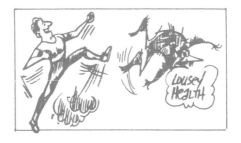

The Simple Art of Nutrition

There are simple, well-defined laws or rules to follow to obtain the utmost from the preparation and use of foods. These laws are natural, easily understood, and readily demonstrated.

Only when we follow these laws and live within their simplicity does our blood become pure and our minds serene. As we live within these simple laws we can dismiss all thoughts of disease, and it will never be necessary to seek help or relief from any outside source.

This excellent health has been achieved in thousands of cases involving every variety of disease condition. All diseases and adverse conditions respond and disappear as we discover the healthy way.

Cleansing, building, and retaining is the master plan of this simple form of nutrition. Before building and retaining can be realized, cleansing of the various toxins, poisons, and congestions must be complete.

I offer you the finest in the cleansing and healing field in the form of the lemonade diet.

In an article in the **National Enquirer,** July 22, 1975, there was the following prediction by Jeanne Dixon: "One of the greatest medical breakthroughs of the decade will come from the common citrus fruit. Scientists will create fantastic new wonder drugs from these fruits for a wide array of illnesses that have plagued mankind for centuries. It will be learned that a chemical in the fruit can strengthen our natural resistance to many diseases."

In reality, the chemical or chemicals present in the citrus do not actually make the body resistant to disease; rather, they eliminate the causes of disease by their cleansing action. These fantastic new wonder chemicals have already been discovered many years ago by me, and they are already being used in the form of the lemonade diet with tremendous success around the world.

There is no need to further create these chemicals as God has already done a better job of it than any group of men can ever hope to do, regardless of their education or abilities. These chemicals are already in the citrus fruit to function at the highest level of efficiency because other necessary chemicals are present with them. As various chemicals are separated or isolated, unbalances, resulting in harmful side effects can occur, defeating the original plan to cleanse and build. Only when we use the best of foods in their **original form,** are we going to get the most out of them.

For many years I have been telling my students that we always need the whole product instead of the various separated units such as carrot juice, vegetable juices, etc. We throw away the pulp — fiber — and take only the juice. There are many needed properties in the fiber also to assist in properly handling the juices. Is it not feasable that the lack of them can cause deficiences or unbalances? We know from excellent results that carrot juice, celery juice and other vegetable juices are excellent but how much better can they be if left intact and taken as is. Can we possibly get as much good and complete nutrition from drinking a dozen carrots without the fiber as we can from properly chewing the whole carrot and eating fewer carrots.

Recent findings tell us that fiber "is that important". Formerly we were told not to use fiber as it might cause a variety of colon troubles. In determining this importance and putting it to use should we go over board with the idea by using such things as wood fiber in bread, (good for termites but not much good for us) or say cereal, or perhaps some other foreign matter in these products or should we use it as it is originally without separating it in the first place. Reminds me of the white bread controversy — tests showed that white bread could not sustain life even though milk and eggs had been added so a variety of vitamins were added — enriched — fortified flour they called it. Then new standards were found or believed to be necessary so more enrichments were added — then extra iron — extra spoilage retardants or preservatives appeared necessary — next extra fiber was found that important. Now after all these things were added just how good was the bread — taking things out and adding other things to replace them. Could they be as good as the original ingredients? White bread has always seemed like a sickly looking mess to me. Surely there is a reason for the bulk and other things being there originally. Perhaps they figured God made a mistake so man must correct it.

The whole matter could have been prevented by leaving things as they were originally. Now if we can accept the whole procedure as a much needed lesson we can then leave the rest of our food as it is and stop taking extra wheat germ, lecithin, vitamins, minerals, fiber (bran or wood) and many other extras to supplement and enrich a large variety of separated and devitalized products.

Another thought by so many people "If a small amount is good: then logic tells them that a lot can do so much more". By taking a lot more isn't it possible that again we might be going overboard and consuming more than the body can handle at one time so we must then work overtime to handle and eliminate the excess or hopelessly clog up the works and defeat our original reason for following the procedures. Then there is the pulp — bulk — which is left out. Something is left out so what deficiences have we created and what about the following side effects?

It seems to me we should start all over again from the beginning: start eating things as they are in limited amounts to allow the body to digest and assimilate just the amount it can handle with no excesses.

The use of a high protein for weight reducing became a fad and then a predigested protein is creating many serious deficiencies and developed a monster to the point that it was reported that many have died from lack of potassium, and other needed life qualities.

This simple idea can and will save us a lot of time, money and useless research to test for possible deficiences. Certainly the monetary saving advantages can become a major importance.

The ideal purpose of any complete diet is to have all the vitamins, minerals, and nutrients in a readily available form in order to enable the body to function normally and to be free from diseases and other malfunctions.

Since many people of the world are already handicapped by a multiplicity of diseases, they must first cleanse the body before the right diet can be properly used. Thus, the sick and suffering must first turn to the best of all cleansing diets, THE MASTER CLEANSER or LEMONADE DIET.

What About the Use of Vitamins?

Vitamins and minerals have always been a necessary part of natural living. Not satisfied with God's plan, man has attempted to improve the situation by separating them from fresh live foods, then processing and combining them to conform to his concept of what they should be. Not satisfied with the finished product, attempts were made to produce them synthetically. It was big business — and we became a world of "pill pushers," whether they were needed or not. More often they were not needed. No one really knew if the pills were needed, or how many — people just took them because they **might** have a deficiency!

Just how these vitamins and minerals should be balanced and formulated led to many differences of opinion. A large variety of experts, in processing and manufacturing of pills, disagree as to how the many billions of pills should be made. They all have different formulas and claim theirs are the best even though much is lost in the processing. However, even without any clear consensus as to their worth and use, they were manufactured and processed; therefore they must be sold with no thought as to possible side effects from overdosing or imbalances. Millions of dollars are made by the producers and the sellers with little regard for the true needs of the consumer.

In reality, the whole process could have been completely avoided. Our Creator has already done a better job of making sure we receive all the needed vitamins and minerals in a perfectly balanced form. Only the finest of natural foods in their original package are good enough for bringing complete energy and life to build and retain a healthy body. Any time man attempts to improve on God's formulas and plans, the result is bound to be a failure.

The simple rules to complete nutrition include all the vitamins and minerals needed by all mankind and all animals. Our Creator has given the right food for the right animal for complete nutrition. This is also true for man. When these foods are properly prepared and eaten, there is nothing more that man can do to prepare a better food.

As we eat the correct foods without excesses, the body will produce ALL the needed vitamins. Foods grown properly, in complete, mineral-rich soil, will have all the minerals in them. Thus, we have no need for vitamin enriched foods, created synthetically by man, nor for extra minerals.

All refined and devitalized foods must be completely eliminated from our diet. If refined and devitalized foods are eaten, then and only then does man have any need for additional supplements. Just how much and what combination, even with long and complicated tests, will probably never be determined, so this form of unnatural nutrition will always be lacking. Such a plan is a very poor substitute for the right way.

MENU SUGGESTIONS

Our system goes through a cleansing process from twelve midnight until twelve noon, and a building program from twelve noon to twelve midnight. Therefore, what is eaten during these respective periods must be harmonious with the natural processes. The following suggestions take this natural process into account.

BREAKFAST: Nothing more is required by the body than fresh lemonade, fresh orange or grapefruit juice. Occasionally, if one has no desire for even this, try some hot peppermint tea. It gives a clean feeling and is a wonderful tonic.

NOON LUNCH: Lunch may be omitted with no ill effects; many will find a small amount of fruit entirely sufficient. If one desires more, a small vegetable or fruit salad may be eaten. Soup (homemade, vegetarian, of course) or tomato juice, hot or cold, may be taken with vegetable salad. Coconut milk or almond milk may be taken with the fruit salad..

Note: Recipes for coconut and almond milk, and for a number of dressings, are to be found on the following pages.

DINNER (Evening): Simple preparation of dinner involves starting with a vegetable soup, then having two or three vegetables steamed slightly. On other occasions try special dishes such as vegetable stew, various types of brown rice dishes (curried rice, Spanish rice, chop suey and rice), chili beans (made with lima beans or red beans), or any recipe using lentils or garbanzos — but no meat, of course. Vegetarian cutlets, and all similar commercially-produced meat substitute preparations, should be used very, very sparingly, or not at all.

All kinds of berries are an excellent addition for both lunch and dinner.

Change your menu daily. Be sure there is plenty of variety from day to day. Do not over eat — stick to small portions. An occasional mono diet meal is always beneficial such as brown rice with coconut milk and a little maple syrup only, steamed artichokes only, fresh green corn only, watermellon, strawberries, honeydew. Many other single items can readily come to mind.

The accepted idea of five necessary categories of foods daily is quite faulty. It is very time consuming, costly and does not accomplish the desired results that simplification can. Different types of foods have different requirement in time and abilities to properly digest them. Too many combinations often cause a variety of digestive disturbances.

COCONUT MILK

Coconut milk may be used in all recipes calling for milk. Other nut milks are also good. They are superior and preferred to the use of any of the animal milks. Use fresh nuts in preference to canned or grated nuts.

To prepare coconut milk, start with liquefier (blender) ½ full of warm water. Add 2 tbsp. of maple syrup and a dash of salt. (These two ingredients may be left out if not desired.)

As liquefier is running (medium to high speed) add chunks of coconut until container is nearly full. (Dried coconut may be used.)

Strain the pulp from the liquid and use the pulp over again by adding fresh warm water to it in the blender. Strain again, and this time throw the used pulp away.

The coconut milk produced in this fashion makes a tasty, nutritious beverage for children or adults in place of animal milk. A number of delicious drinks can be made by using coconut milk and your favorite fresh fruit liquefied together.

COCONUT-SESAME MILK
(May be used for many cream sauces.)

6 tbsp. grated coconut
6 tbsp. fresh sesame seeds
Sesame or safflower oil

Liquefy the two dry ingredients until they no longer fall to center. Stop the blender and push them to the center with a knife several times as they stick to the sides.

As liquefier is running add sesame or safflower oil until the oil covers the pulp (approx. 6 tbsp.). Liquefy for 2 minutes and then add warm water until mixture reaches the desired thickness (approx. 12 oz. of water). One tbsp. of maple syrup and a dash of salt may be added if desired.

FOR SAUCES: Start with coconut milk, or coconut-sesame milk; add potato flour for thickening and season with desired spices. May also be used for creamed soups (mushroom, celery, etc.) and scalloped dishes (potato, cauliflower, etc.) Try variations as your imagination dictates.

ALMOND MILK

Start with 1 lb. of shelled almonds (dry) in the blender. Blend until they no longer fall to the center. Push them to the center with a knife several times as they stick to the side as the blender is running. Add sesame or safflower oil until pulp is covered (approximately 7 tbsp.) Blend for 2 minutes more and then add warm water until mixture is desired thickness. Two to three glasses of water should be sufficient. One or two tbsp. of maple syrup and a dash of salt may be added if desired.

This makes a nice drink or may be used for any milk recipe.

MAYONNAISE

Start with the coconut-sesame milk, but keep it medium thick by using less than the customary water. Add the following:

5 tbsp. apple cider vinegar
1 tbsp. maple syrup
2 cloves garlic
1 tsp. paprika
1 tsp. chili powder
1 tsp. powdered mustard
1 tsp. turmeric
½ tsp. sweet basil
Salt to taste

FRENCH DRESSING

To the mayonnaise dressing add one good sized tomato or 1 cup tomato juice.

WHITE SAUCE

2 tbsp. margarine or vegetable oil
2 tbsp. potato or brown rice flour
Hot Water

Melt the margarine in a sauce pan. Stir in the potato or rice flour. Continue stirring as you add hot water until you have the desired thickness (approx. 1 cup). Salt as desired.

VARIATIONS OF WHITE SAUCE

1. To the white sauce add 1 tsp. each cardamom and coriander. The cardamon and coriander can be increased — even doubled to improve the taste.
2. Leave out the water and add one 8 oz. can of tomato sauce and ½ tsp. sweet basil.

VEGETABLE SALAD DRESSING No. 1

Using preceding mayonnaise dressing to start add extra spices, delicately, such as dill seed, curry powder, cayenne pepper, fennel seed, or oregano. A couple of dill pickles and sweet relish may be added to provide the Thousand Island taste.

VEGETABLE SALAD DRESSING No. 2

¾ cup olive, sesame, or safflower oil
½ cup vinegar (apple cider or wine)
2 tbsp. lemon or lime juice
3 tbsp. maple syrup
½ tsp. paprika
2 tsp. mustard
1 tsp. sweet basil
1 tsp. dill seed
½ tsp. cardamom
2 cloves garlic
2 tbsp. potato flour (optional)

Blend the oil and vinegar together first with the maple syrup, then add the other ingredients. Add the potato flour as needed if you desire the dressing to be thicker and creamier.

Other herbs and spices may be used very delicately instead of the suggested ones to create a variety of dressings.

COLE SLAW DRESSING No. 1

Start with the basic mayonnaise dressing and add:

1 tsp. dill seed
4 tbsp. vinegar
½ tsp. fennel seed

COLE SLAW DRESSING No. 2

¼ cup oil (cold pressed)
¼ tsp. powdered cloves
¼ tsp. ginger
¼ cup maple syrup
¼ cup apple cider vinegar
Salt
Juice of whole lemon
2 slices pineapple (¾" x 4")
2-3 tbsp. potato flour

Liquefy above ingredients, except potato flour, for 5 minutes. Slowly add potato flour as liquefier is running until desired thickness is achieved.

FRUIT SALAD DRESSING No. 1

Start with the basic coconut-sesame milk, then add:

½ cup maple syrup
2 ripe bananas
1 cup pineapple pieces (fresh if possible)

Nutmeg and cinnamon may be added for extra flavor.

FRUIT SALAD DRESSING No. 2

½ cup water
½ cup maple syrup
4 tbsp. coconut — powdered or fine
2 tbsp. sesame or good oil
½ cup raw cashews or a banana (to thicken)
1 slice fresh pineapple if possible

Cinnamon and nutmeg if desired.
Liquefy for 5 minutes.

The Blessing

Asking God to bless the food before a meal has been an accepted ritual handed down from generation to generation. It has been thought by some to promote better nutrition and healing by raising the vibration of the food.

Better that we ask God to bless our proper selection of more complete foods as we go shopping for that which will advance our physical and our spiritual needs.

Ask Him to bless the preparation of the food, and for temperance in eating, so as to enable our bodies to receive the utmost of value from what God has so abundantly supplied for our daily use.

Ask Him to bless the animal, fish, or fowl we did NOT kill that we may better sustain our lives with the finer qualities of live fresh fruit, vegetables, and seeds.

Better to ask God to give us KNOWLEDGE to keep our bodies strong and healthy so we have no need to ask Him to heal a sick and ailing body that we produced ourselves by not originally obeying His simple laws.

Blame not God for the many illnesses and diseases you have created (they are not "Acts of God"!). Better that you ask God for His blessings and forgiveness — and to give strength and wisdom to properly apply the knowledge of His simple laws.

CHAPTER II:

Vita Flex

Vita Flex is based upon a complete system of internal body "controls." When properly applied to the appropriate "control points", a vibration of healing energy is released to heal, to relieve all pain, and to remove the symptoms as well as the causes of illness. This reflex system of controls encompasses the entire body and mind, releasing all kinds of tensions, congestions, and mal-adjustments.

The standard teachings tell us we have a nervous sytem, a circulatory system, and a bony structure. However, superseding and controlling all the systems (and the mind) is the reflex system not generally recognized by orthodox medicine. It even extends into the Physic. It is a life force or healing energy which is capable of producing fast corrections of illness with an effectiveness such as no other method can even approximate.

There is a similarity between Vita Flex and the ancient art of Acupuncture. It has been known and used in many parts of India and the Orient as Acupressure; in this form, finger pressure is applied rather than the inserting of needles. The Vita Flex system works similar to a computer made by man only more efficiently and more accurately. You might consider it as having a Divine intelligence within us that works automatically, constantly on the alert, constantly making repairs, corrections, necessary changes, growing, eliminating the old to rebuild with new.

This computer works automatically to cover all our needs if we in turn give it complete co-operation by eating and living to the best of our ability by the simple natural laws of complete living. Each time we go counter to these natural laws the computer will make every attempt to correct or rebalance the error.

As a woman becomes pregnant and the baby is being formed; consciously she does not start giving directions as to where the eyes are to be placed or how they are to be made or where the limbs are to be placed or made. She simply goes on with normal living and the Divine intelligence within her automatically designs and builds the body to a perfect specimen.

That does not mean that she can ignore her part in the process. She must eat properly and live within certain well defined natural laws of living. Even then the automatic system often compensates for any negligence on the part of the mother. If she does not supply all the necessary nutrition in the food she eats or if she consumes various toxic foods or drinks the computer or Divine intelligence will often take from the mother nourishment for the baby. Clean out the body to protect the baby or when extreme deficiencies or many toxins exist then the baby may be born with various deformities. It is up to us to make it possible for this automatic computer to have the supply it needs to function with the utmost efficiency.

To further help this computer to function normally we are provided with control points (keys or buttons) all over the body. This is Vita Flex — a complete set of controls. Each time the control points are pressed there is an electric spark of energy which goes to an exact point. When it reaches this point necessary changes are made automatically.

The true and complete knowledge of this work can only be found in the system I have developed over many years of research and experimentation, and which I present here under the name of Vita Flex. This entire work is done without the need for anything more than just the fingers. It works faster and more completely than systems employing needles. Since so many people object to having needles stuck into various parts of the body, Vita Flex is more readily accepted by the general public. It takes a much longer time to correctly place a number of needles — wait, twist, and then place more in other parts. The Vita Flex way moves fast to effect the entire body quickly, accurately, and more effectively. Results achieved occur in a small fraction of the time required by other systems and hence involve far lower cost.

There are more than five thousand Vita Flex points of control compared to only three hundred sixty-five acupuncture points as usually taught. With Vita Flex the affected parts are never treated directly, but rather on reflected points, thus not causing further injury to the damaged part.

Many years of research have led me to the discovery that this system apparently originated in Tibet many thousands of years ago; long before Acupuncture was discovered.

It has been a tremendous pleasure of accomplishment to revive this ancient art, to bring people healing in its simplest and most effective form. It is a type of healing which has absolutely no dangerous or destructive side effects. Only positive and direct healing takes place at any time.

This system completely eliminates the need for costly and lengthy tests, diagnosis, and observations. Many long hours and days of tedious and often painful traction are completely unnecessary, for this method works within minutes. A large variety of conditions disappear long before any form of diagnosis can determine the name of the disease. Most of the need for X-rays is eliminated.

Perhaps one of the most valuable accomplishments in this system is the extremely low cost involved. The cost of orthodox medical care has grown by leaps and bounds, making the whole procedure complicated, archaic, and beyond the reach of many patients.

Vita Flex simply means vitality through the reflexes. It is a complete, scientific, workable system of controls which releases the energy of the unlimited healing powers within us.

It is applied to various key points all over the body by a pressure with a pull of the finger and a slight twist of the wrist. The twist increases the leverage and pressure on the points of contact. It is similar to the action of a pipe wrench. The more you twist it the tighter and more effective it becomes. As the twist continues to completion, the finger is completely bent and the correct pressure actually occurs with the end of the finger making the contact. All this time, the hand remains firm on the foot, hand or other part of the body with no slipping. The final pressure is medium to heavy. The pressure is never held, but released immediately and repeated from the beginning. This may be done several times on the same spot as required to obtain desired results.

Since this system is very fast, one will never stay more than a moment on any point, thus preventing unnecessary irritations. Do not rub on any point as this rubbing can do a lot of damage to the tissues. Since we are not attempting to crush crystals, which may or may not be there,

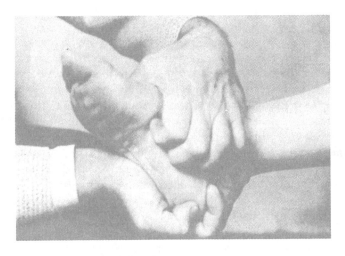

No. 1   Note curl of first finger

we use the pipe wrench technique — a pressure and a release. As the progress continues on to other parts, the hand moves smoothly and rhythmically without jerks and jabs. Do not jerk in doing any of the reflex work at any time. Jerking can harm a person. The application of pressure is applied with either one of the first two fingers and occasionally the thumb, and must be specific, on the exact point, done exactly right. Fingers may be switched from time to time as they get tired. The finger nails must be cut and smooth to the lowest possible point. (Note No. 1 the first finger of the left hand.)

There are many reflex actions taking place from the same control point to many other areas, as well as the designated spot. This will be explained from time to time as we come to these points.

This advanced method works instantaneously, thus eliminating any need of prolonged crushing massage that might damage the tissues. Pressure to reflexes of the entire body may be completed in a relatively short period. There is no need to remove any part of the clothing except the shoes. Socks may actually be left on to advantage. The entire work is thus so simple that it may be used at any time and in any place.

The possibilities this system brings to mind are unlimited. In the field of First Aid there is nothing that can compare with it. Scout Masters may relieve all types of pain from sprains, twists, dislocations, cramps, fevers, and indigestion. Many more conditions respond to this marvelous science. And what applies to Scout Masters can also apply to you in any and all emergencies.

No piece of machinery made by man, no matter how wonderful it is, can compare with the mechanism that the Creator gave to us in this beautiful body of ours. As He gave us this body, He also gave us a complete system of controls that make it possible to keep the body in perfect running order, if we will but follow the rules. **We become sick to the same extent to which we ignore these rules.**

From the very beginning of man's existence, he has, knowingly or unknowingly, used this system of pain relief. With primitive man, living close to Nature, he walked or ran from place to place either barefooted or with thin foot covering. Thus he stepped on sticks or stones and in so doing, he automatically pressed and stimulated various reflexes. As he used his hands in work or play, again he activated the reflexes. Modern man may now use this complete arrangement of reflex controls, which are found all over the body, to give fast relief. The stimulation is applied from the outside, but remember, the healing process takes place within.

There are seven or more control points for each affected part. These points may be used as often as desired as long as the skin or flesh is not injured. They may be used several times a day as needed to remove pain and to prompt the body to heal itself.

The reflex system stimulates or depresses only to a normal condition. There are no dangerous side effects.

The Four Dimensions of Vita Flex

With Vita Flex, we work through four dimensions, three of which are literal, geographical dimensions. One dimension goes up and down (from head to toe and reverse) another straight across (from side to side) and the third straight through (from front to back and reverse). Each one works independently, yet all four dimensions work together for complete action.

First Dimension

As you look at the bottom of the feet, picture both as representing the body from the hips up. The outer part of the feet represents the outer part of the body. Example: The reflexes on the outer part of the right foot affect the outer right side of the body and the head. The reflexes on the outer part of the left foot affect the outer left side of the body and head. The inner part of the feet represent the spine and center of the body, while the heels represent the hips and the toes represent the head. The above also applies to the hands. Thus, in miniature, the feet and hands represent the entire body.

There are many control points in between the head and feet that also go both up and down. For a sprained or injured ankle, relief is found by working the corresponding part on the wrist of the same side. The bottom of the foot is also for the ankle (same side). For wrist conditions, work on the corresponding part of the ankle on the same side. The palm of the hand is also used for the wrist. Cramps or pains in the calf of the legs are relieved by working on the forearm. For arm pains, work the same area of the legs on the same side. The same is true of the elbows and knees and all other parts in the legs and arms. For pain in the feet, work on the corresponding part of the hand on the same side. There is one exception, however, in this principle. For a pain in the hand, go to the reflexes directly above the elbow, both front and back. Reflexes directly below the elbow go to the upper arm and shoulder. Reflexes directly above the knee caps go downward to the feet and ankles. Reflexes directly below the knee cap go to the upper part of the legs and hips.

Second Dimension

The Second Dimension is straight across. The entire half of either side is a complete reflex to the corresponding opposite side. Example: Pain in one ankle may be relieved by the reflexes in the opposite ankle. One knee relieves pain in the other knee. So it is for the legs, hips, back, shoulders, arms, hands, and head.

Third Dimension

The Third Dimension covers the entire body from the front to the back and reverse. Example: Headaches in the front of the head may be relieved by working on the reflex points on the back of the head and vice versa. Body pains in front are relieved by going to the exact spot in back. The same method for pains in the back.

Fourth Dimension

There is but one body and but one spirit. We are all an extension, or expression, of the Divine. We are all connected together with cords visible only through the spiritual sight. What affects one, affects the whole world and all its people. What we do to ourselves, we do to others. What we do to others, we do to ourselves.

There are four methods by which the Fourth Dimension in healing others works. The first method is to work the Vita Flex system on one's self. The part of the body that is effected can be relieved or healed by the duplicate part or parts being worked on. Example: A person may have a pain in the hip. The operator works **on his own hip** with the Vita Flex principle and while doing this he visualizes himself as actually working on the person. As the operator does this, the correction is made on the other person. The second method works by working through another person (a third party) while still visualizing working on the person with the pain. The third method works by picturing mentally the affected area of the person. Visualize yourself actually working on the diseased spot or spots. The fourth method is done by working mentally on the mind of the person; visualize the person's own mind doing the healing directly. These all work according to an automatic law which is ours to use as we need it to help raise mankind to his rightful heritage of perfection in health.

As you work knowingly with these laws, they will work for you, provided your desire to heal is sincere and completely honest. Do not attempt to use any of these powers just for entertainment or experimental purposes. They are only for the select in the advanced healing field.

These fourth dimension healing forces work whether the person is right in the room or thousands of miles away. Space is not a handicap. These healing forces work with no regard to the ordinary conception of time. The operator may project healing to any individual at any time and mentally direct it to happen at another time on another day and it will take place at that time only.

These healing forces may be directed to one individual or group of individuals just as the operator desires. Each person in the group of individuals receives an equal amount of the healing power.

Please do not attempt to use any part of the fourth dimension by itself until the other three are thoroughly and completely understood. Even when more experienced, do not use the fourth dimension by itself except in extreme emergencies. **Work all dimensions together for the best results.**

44

The entire system works whether one believes in it or not. It works by scientific methods, not by faith. The skeptics may also be healed. Belief and faith offers a higher vibration, however, and thus quicker action.

The true secret of the art of healing is to understand that everything has its own rate of vibration. The various forms of disease have their own rate — thus we appear to have a large variety of diseases. These vibrations are of different levels but they are all below the level of health.

By using all four dimensions in the physical, mental, and spiritual field, our vibrations are raised to the higher levels and health replaces disease. Changing the vibrations replaces the many errors of tests, diagnosis, medication, operations and excessive costs of an archaic and destructive system. Complete freedom from all diseases is a lifetime reality.

The Spinal Reflexes

All spine conditions can be corrected by the reflex system. By applying Vita Flex to the feet and hands, it is possible for the entire spine to be adjusted to its correct position. In No. 4 and No. 2 you will note that on

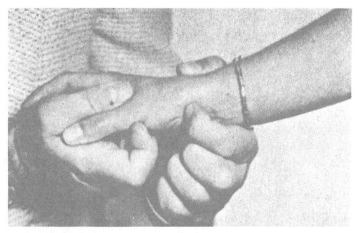

No. 4   Reflexes of the spine

the hand the distance of approximately one inch takes in the reflexes of the entire spine. The reflex closest to the thumb is the atlas or top of the spine, while the reflex by the wrist is the tail bone. Pain in any part of the spine may be relieved by applying reflex action to the corresponding point. Similarly with the feet, on the inner edge of the arch close to the bunion joint are found the reflexes to the top of the spine, and at the opposite end of the arch is the tail bone. (No. 5) The right hand and foot control the right side of the spine and the left hand and foot control the left side.

PALM OF RIGHT HAND

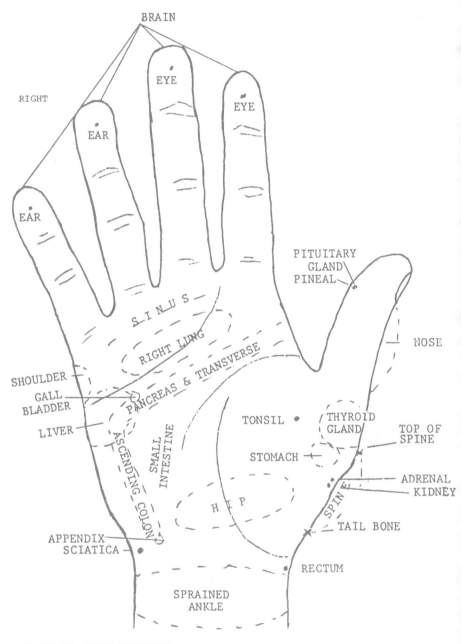

WORK ON CORRESPONDING
PART OF HAND TO RELIEVE
PAIN IN FOOT

46

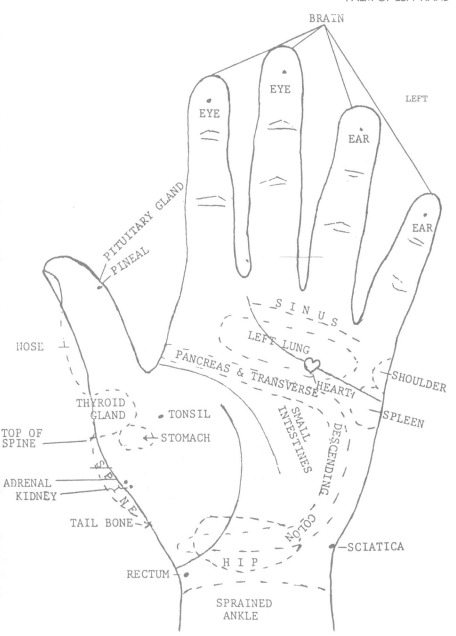

PALM OF LEFT HAND

BRAIN

EYE

EYE

LEFT

EYE

EAR

EAR

PITUITARY GLAND

PINEAL

S I N U S

LEFT LUNG

NOSE

PANCREAS & TRANSVERSE

HEART

SHOULDER

THYROID GLAND

TONSIL

SMALL INTESTINES

DESCENDING

SPLEEN

TOP OF SPINE

STOMACH

ADRENAL
KIDNEY

S P I N E

TAIL BONE

COLON

SCIATICA

HIP

RECTUM

SPRAINED
ANKLE

WORK ON CORRESPONDING
PART OF HAND TO RELIEVE
PAIN IN FOOT

47

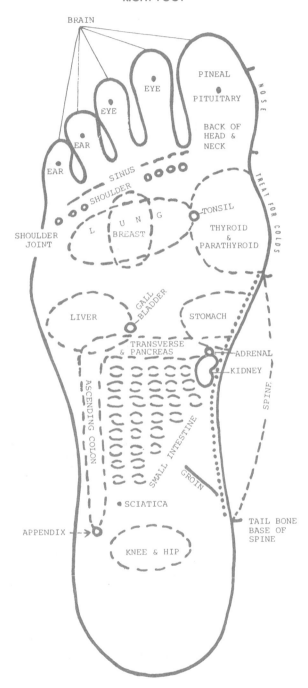

RIGHT FOOT

LEFT FOOT

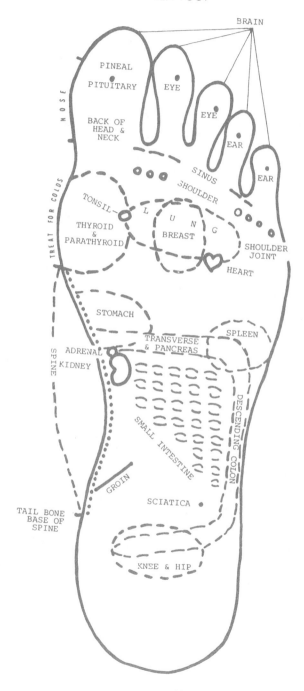

49

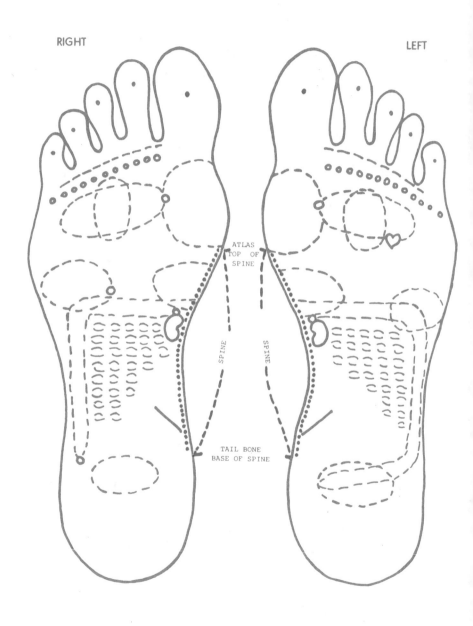

RIGHT

LEFT

ATLAS
TOP OF
SPINE

SPINE

SPINE

TAIL BONE
BASE OF SPINE

The tail bone and atlas corrections are often made with the first treatment. Stiff and sore muscles, beside the spine, relax and loosen. Various curvatures respond rapidly for complete correction.

Formerly, a crushed or cracked disk had no means of correction. Direct manipulation or massage could cause dangerous injury. With Vita Flex, these corrections can be made painlessly in about seven daily treatments.

A simple explanation of the adjustment process is demonstrated with a ruler. Center the ruler on the first finger. This represents the fulcrum. The finger would represent the spine. By placing a coin on one end of the ruler, it becomes unbalanced. To rebalance again, the ruler must be moved to change the fulcrum. Nature never tolerates an imbalance, so automatically, changes are made when these imbalances occur.

Since Vita Flex works through the reflected area, rather than the affected, no injury can occur. Herein lies the secret of Vita Flex. The science of automatic precision throughout the body produces the necessary correction. Through these reflex points, we contact the controlling power of the spine.

The Colon (Constipation)
(No. 6)

As the waste matter passes from the small intestine into the colon, the appendix discharges a lubrication for better elimination. The appendix is a very necessary part of our eliminative process and must not be taken out. Any congestion settling there may be broken up without removing

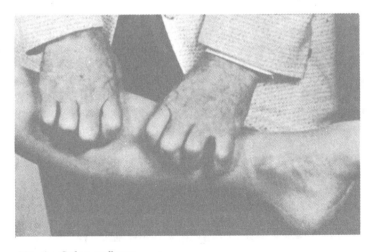

No. 6   Colon reflexes

51

it. Complete action for proper elimination starts with the peristaltic action at the appendix on the right foot. Start the reflex action at this point. From there, continue up the side of the foot to the liver. This is the ascending colon. From the liver, continue directly across the right foot **and on to the left** — continue across the left to the spleen. Work with both hands back and forth over this area as this will take in the transverse colon and the pancreas. From the spleen continue down the side of the left foot. This is the descending colon. As the heel is reached, work across the foot to the tail bone reflex. This completes the circuit of the colon.

Reflexes along the full length of the inner part of both shin bones relieves gas and congestion in the colon. Work up under the bone. (No. 6).

I am strongly opposed to colonics or enemas as they can do much damage. Only in extreme emergencies, should this action be taken. After the emergency has passed, then Nature can be helped to normal elimination. A mild herb laxative tea is best for a temporary help. A good program of exercise or Yoga is by far the best.

Working on the reflexes to all parts of the colon, liver, pancreas, and spleen stimulates and activates the natural secretions of insulin for the permanent correction of diabetes. Of course, the correct food must be eaten as given in the Master Cleanser — see page 13 for further information on diabetes.

The Stomach

(No's 7, 8, 9 and 10)

The basic cause of all diseases is the toxins that produce congestion, which in turn block the natural functions of the body. These toxins clog or delay the many automatic controls. If the body does not have proper material to work with, it cannot build effectively or throw off the waste matter fast enough.

The stomach becomes our first organ to suffer from our dietary mistakes, and often with the painful disorder known as an ulcer. Ulcers are not caused by nerves but by incorrect and deficient diet. The wall of the stomach is coated with sodium which protects it from being digested by the digestive juices. Flesh foods of all kinds attract sodium. As we eat these foods, the sodium is drawn from the wall of the stomach and surrounds the meat, making it indigestible in the stomach. It must be broken down in the intestines. (The least harmful way of eating flesh food is to swallow it in chunks as a dog does — this manner leaves less surface for the attraction of sodium.) Through the extensive use of meat, particularly if not coupled with the eating of high sodium content foods, one finds too late that there is no protective stomach coating left. In this condition the stomach proceeds to digest itself and the result is known as an ulcer.

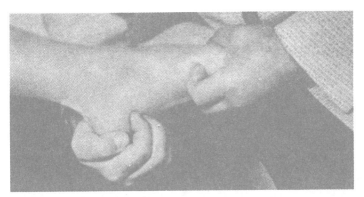

No. 7   Left hand shows stomach reflexes

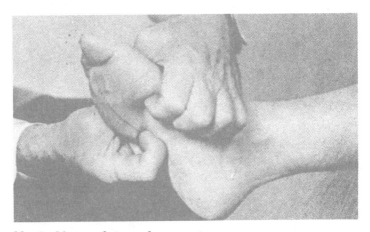

No. 8   Liver and stomach

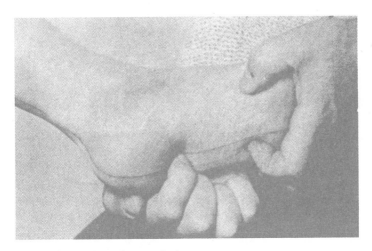

No. 9   Stomach, spleen, sciatica

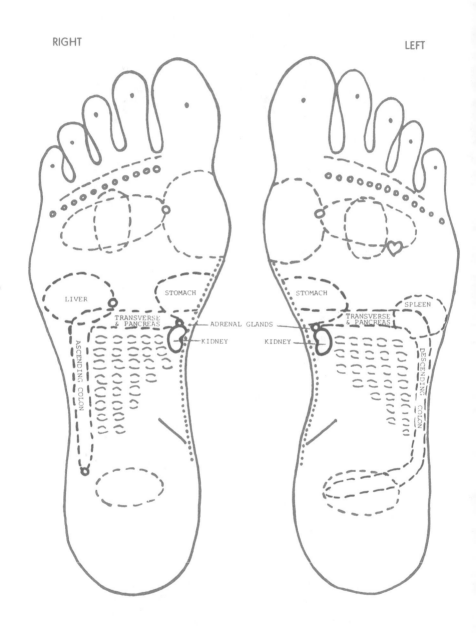

RIGHT

LEFT

LIVER

STOMACH

STOMACH

SPLEEN

TRANSVERSE
& PANCREAS

TRANSVERSE
& PANCREAS

ADRENAL GLANDS

KIDNEY

KIDNEY

ASCENDING COLON

DESCENDING COLON

The reflexes to the stomach are found just below the bunion joint on the bottom of each foot. The right foot reflexes are for the outlet of the stomach; the left foot reflexes are for the inlet to the stomach. Other stomach reflexes are below the second joint on the thumbs and on the top part of the upper arms.

Prolapsed Organs

Devitalized and toxic diets of this modern civilization, abetted by the absence of simple stretching and strengthening exercises and the constant presence of gravity have produced serious prolapses of the organs in many people. The abdominal organs have simply slipped downward into a heap in the bottom of the abdominal cavity, restricting the area blood supply.

The colon has many minute pockets and by eating devitalized foods these pockets become filled with hardened wastes causing gas and constipation. Though one may begin to eat wholesome food, without muscular toning exercises or some method of restoring the organs to their proper position, even good nutrients are prevented from building the body as they should.

By observing the foot chart, Pages 42 & 43, you will note that the transverse colon in proper position, extends straight across the abdomen just below the waist line. When prolapsed it will curve downward in various positions.

For making corrections of this prolapsed condition it is necessary to have a slanting board with a strap to hold the feet on the higher end.

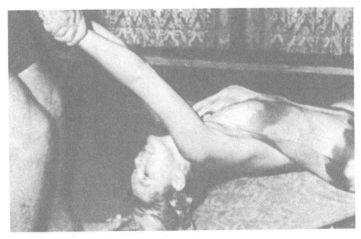

No. 11   Prolapsed organs

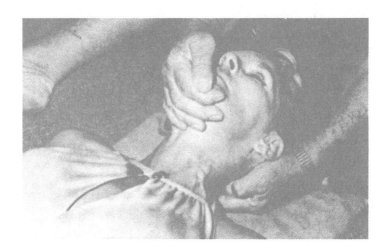

No. 12   Prolapsed organs

The person being treated lies on his back on the slant board with head down and feet hooked under the straps. Stretch the arms over the head — there will be a pleasant relaxing of the spine. Further stretching may be done by grasping the wrist of the person and pulling at the same time, allowing the head to drop down as in No. 11. (No. 12).

The assistant should carefully check over the various areas from the pelvic bone to the ribs for extreme tenderness, then gradually knead as if working on rising bread dough. This should be done for 10 to 15 minutes to help break up adhesions and congestions. (No. 13 and 14).

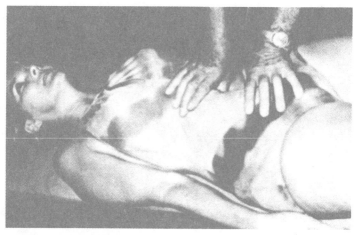

No. 13   Prolapsed organs

56

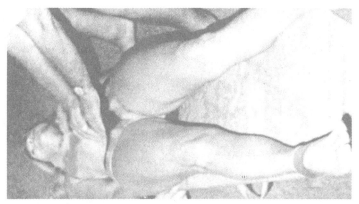

No. 14   Prolapsed organs

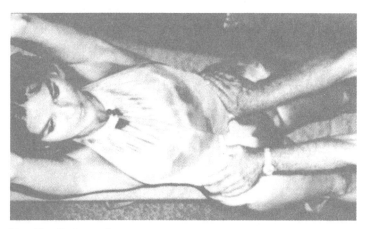

No. 15   Prolapsed organs

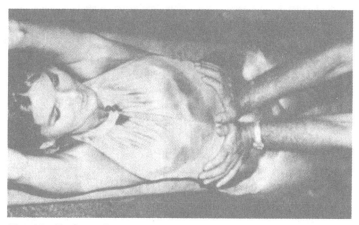

No. 16   Prolapsed organs

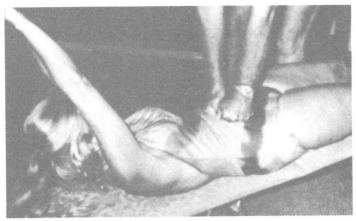

No. 17   Prolapsed organs

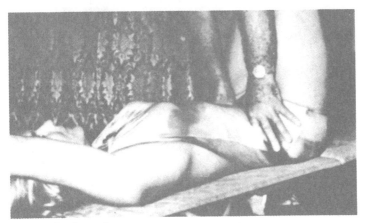

No. 18   Prolapsed organs

From time to time, as tension or lumps are found in the area, the corresponding reflex points of the feet should be worked on. These tensions, lumps, or congestions quickly disappear and further exploration and massage should continue in all the pelvic and intestinal areas.

Next, starting at the pelvic bone, press downward with the thumbs and heel of the hands as far as is reasonably possible and exert pressure upward toward the ribs at the same time. (No. 15). This should be repeated several times, moving closer toward the ribs each time. This series of pushes with pressure gradually raises the organs to their original position. To keep them there, start with the thumbs and heel of the hands again on the pelvic bone. Press down, and at the same time have the person raise the arms, head, and shoulders up high enough to make the muscles push the thumbs and heel of the hands up. (No. 16 and 17). Do this 7 or 8 times. Repeat the same exercise, but this time have the person raise both feet slowly until they are perpendicular to the body

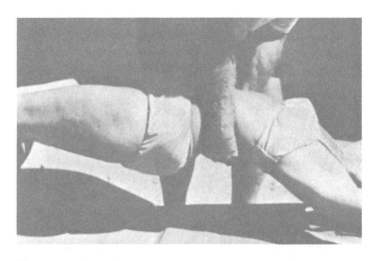

No. 19   Prolapsed organs

without bending the knees. (No. 18). Before the legs are lowered, have the person relax and draw the diaphragm in as far as possible and hold in that position as the legs are lowered:

To complete the uplift, the assistant may hold the subject firmly in the lower part of the back and lift high enough to form an arch. The subject may be raised up and down several times in this manner shaking them slightly each time. This exercise stretches and relaxes the entire back. (No. 19).

Modern civilization, with its devitalized food and minimal exercise, has left a large majority of the people needing the abdominal organ uplift for better digestion, assimilation, and elimination. When all organs are in their right place, every part functions more efficiently. Underweight persons put on needed weight more readily and obese conditions are overcome more readily when all functions operate normally. The uplift also helps to relieve pressure on the pelvic organs for menstral cramps and painless child birth.

To keep the organs in place, one should continue sit ups and leg lifts every day for at least 15 minutes with a bag of about 25 pounds of sand on the stomach and intestinal area.

No. 20   Reflex points for high and low blood pressure

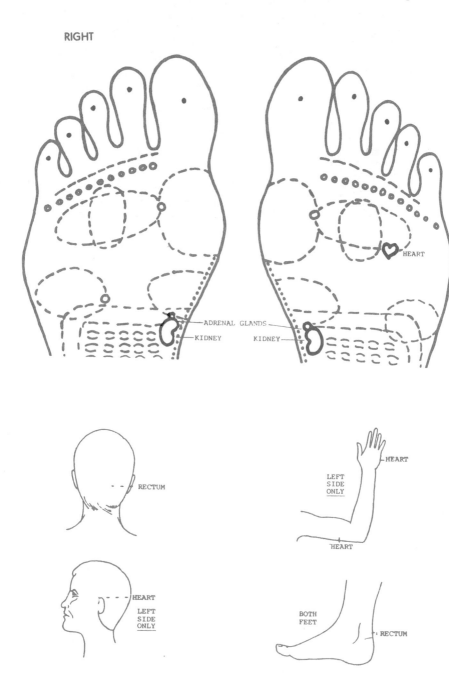

RIGHT

HEART

ADRENAL GLANDS
KIDNEY
KIDNEY

RECTUM

HEART
LEFT
SIDE
ONLY

HEART
LEFT
SIDE
ONLY

HEART
BOTH
FEET
RECTUM

Heart and Blood Pressure Controls

There are two types of blood pressure: the Systolic, during which time the heart cavities contract and force the blood onward; the Diastolic, during which time the heart cavities expand and fill with blood. Normal blood pressure is 120 over 75 for persons of any age.

There are four main reflexes to the heart, to raise or lower the **Systolic** to a normal condition:

- The heart reflex in the left foot slows the heart and makes the beat stronger. (No. 20).
- The reflexes in the left hand, and in the arm above the elbow, make the heart beat regular. (No. 21). Use your right hand to work on the heart reflex in the left hand. Use your left hand to work on the heart reflex in the left arm. First work on the reflex for the heart on the left hand and then on the arm, back to the hand and continue alternating the action.

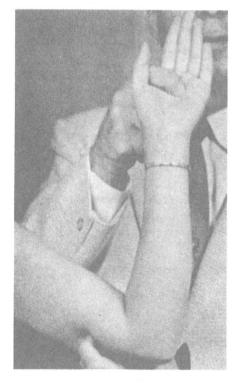

No. 21 Reflex points for heart

61

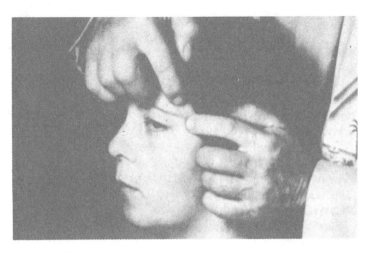

No. 22   Heart and sciatic

- Near the left eye is the reflex to make the heart beat faster and stronger. (No. 22).

To raise or lower the **Diastolic** pressure, the reflexes to the kidneys, adrenal glands, and rectum are used. These points are found on both the feet and the head. (No. 20).

To control fainting or heart attacks, start with the heart reflex in the left hand and arm, then switch to the reflex on the head near the eye. All points should be worked on until normal conditions return.

There have been many instances of a person pronounced dead being brought back to life while the reflexes to the heart are being worked on.

These reflexes work fast to revive a person after drowning. It is a better and faster way than mouth to mouth resuscitation or rhythmic pressure on the lungs.

The Eyes and Ears

The following control points are for the immediate relief of all headaches. For best results all of them may be used, but usually only a few are needed. The fastest relief points are in both elbows, (No. 23), the reflex points for the top of the spine and stomach in both thumbs, and two points at the back of the head. (No. 26 and 24). These same points also release tension and pain across both shoulders and around the neck area. Other eye and ear reflexes are found in the center of the pads of all toes and fingers. The ends of the toes and fingers relieve aches on top of

62

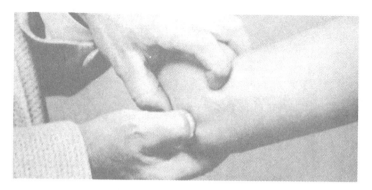

No. 23   Eye and ear

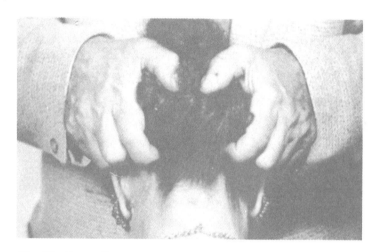

No. 24   Eye reflexes

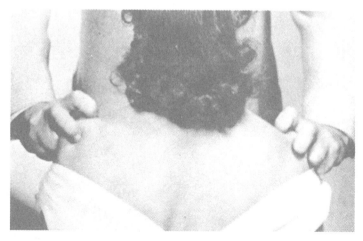

No. 25   Eye and ear reflexes

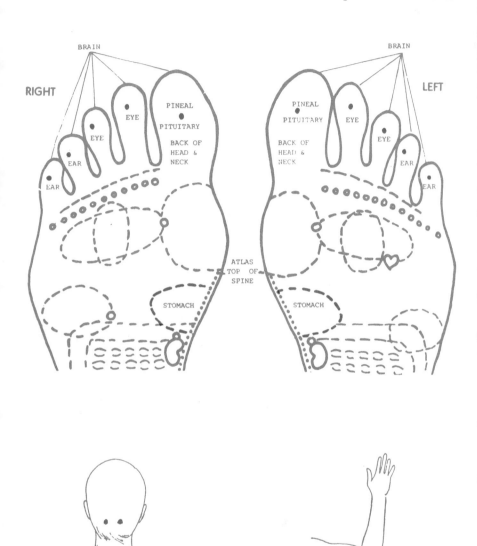

the head and brain. It is rare that these finger and toe reflex points are needed for headaches, but they are important for helping other eye and ear problems. (No. 25 and 29).

The pituitary gland controls are also important relief points for headaches. These points are found in the center of the first joint pads of both thumbs and big toes. These points stimulate or depress the pituitary to normal function. This is the Master gland. When this is functioning to full activity, the rest of the body becomes in tune with it. The worst of all headaches and sinus problems have always responded to this system in seconds. Often they are gone permanently. Those returning may again be relieved at any time and as often as needed. This system works when other forms of treatment or drugs fail completely — there isn't a drug on the market that can compare with its fast results. And they are accomplished with no side effects or hangovers. There is no longer a need to live with this form of pain, or any other pain, when an entire system is available to eliminate the causes.

Special Formula for Eye Drops

This formula has been used with most excellent results for many years with absolutely no dangerous side effects when coupled with a change of diet, the reflex work, and color therapy. Many cases of glaucoma, cataracts, spots, film, and growths of various kinds have completely disappeared. The drops may be applied one at a time to both eyes several times daily. Continue use until the condition is cleared up. Many people have completely overcome the necessity for glasses. In all cases eyes have improved greatly. There are a number of books written on eye exercises; their systems help greatly to bring the sight back to normal. Most people would do well to learn and perform exercises to insure the retention of normal vision.

Formula: 5 parts (measures) distilled water
2 parts best grade of honey
1 part pure apple cider vinegar
(Sterling or other good brand)

Mix together and store in a bottle. It need not be refrigerated as contents will not spoil. If eyes are in good condition, keep them that way by regular use as no harm can ever come by using it. It has a strong smarting effect for a moment, then the eyes clear and feel very good after each use. These drops have proven to be superior to most commercial drops.

Respiratory Conditions

Asthma, hay fever, sinus, pneumonia, TB, emphysema, and other breathing problems are controlled as follows:

The thyroid and parathyroid glands control the breathing. The thyroid gland controls the air coming into the lungs (inhalation) and the parathyroid gland controls the air going out of the lungs (exhalation). They act like a pump working in opposition to each other. Both glands are found in the throat extending from the center toward both sides of the neck. The controls for these glands are found around the bunion joint of both toes. Start with the kidney reflexes (on both feet), then the bunion joints. Work on the top, side and bottom, and all the way around. Next the outer side of the big toes for the nose; then pituitary glands in the center of the first joint pads on both large toes; finally the bronchial tubes (found on top of feet between and directly below the joints of the big toes and the first toes). The tonsil reflexes are found on the bottom of the feet directly below the bronchial reflexes. Working all around the big toes (side, bottom and tops) also relieves tension and head aches in back of head. Next work (with all fingers placed at the base of the toes on both feet) on sinus points closing fists and bending toes down to create more pressure on the points. Use the same method to work on the lung reflexes but just slightly below. (No. 28).

The reflex point for the bronchial tubes also correct pain or congestion in the back, directly back of the bronchial tubes. (No. 27).

No. 27   Reflex to bronchial tubes

RIGHT

LEFT

67

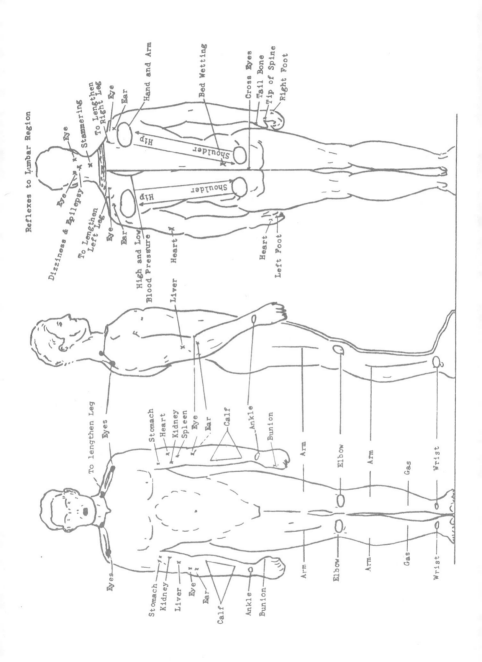

Adjusting The Legs
(No. 29 and 30)

Many disorders, aches and pains in the back, hips, spine and neck originate in the maladjustment of the hips and atlas. A large percentage of the people have one leg shorter than the other. To make this correction, the atlas must be in normal position. Few systems of healing have any knowledge of how to make this correction, so they build up the heel or place a pad in the heel of the short leg. Those who have been partially successful in making the correction take much time and many treatments — as fast as the correction is made the condition frequently returns and must be corrected over and over again.

The Vita-Flex system has the immediate answer. The first adjustment makes a complete correction that will rarely go out of place again. If such a situation does happen, instant correction is made again by this method. The person being treated must be seated squarely and evenly on the chair. The person making the change stands in back of the patient and another may hold the feet up slightly to watch the change. The control points for this correction are found in the collar bone on both sides. As the collar bone comes from the front of the throat and extends out across the shoulders, there is a slightly projected point at the turn. By placing the thumb on this point and rolling, inwardly; around and under it, the correction is made. The pressure must be quite strong and deep. If the change does not take place immediately, either you are missing the spot or the pressure is not strong enough.

To properly make the change, the thumb is first pressed on the side of the short leg. This may be done several times. If the leg is still short, then

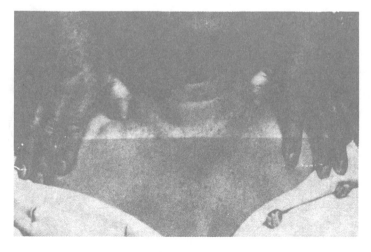

No. 30   Reflex points to lengthen legs

use the same pressure on the other side and the long leg shortens to make both legs even. It is interesting and exciting to watch the short leg move down to the same length as the other, as the adjustment is being made.

After the correction is made, or if no correction is needed, further pressure will never alter the condition, in an adverse way.

Usually, one leg is not really shorter than the other. It only appears so because the hip and atlas are out of place. Because the pelvic bone is tipped higher on one side, the leg on that side is shorter. If a bone in one leg is really shorter than the other side due to an accident or a form of disease, there is no pretense of lengthening the bone to make the correction.

Shoulder Disorders
(No. 31)

Arthritis, bursitis, rheumatism, neuritis and similar conditions all develop from the same source — incorrect food that produces toxins. Refer to the Master Cleanser for more detail. (See page 10).

Pains in the shoulder joint (bursitis) are relieved and corrected at the phalangeal joint at the base of the little toes and little fingers. For soreness or congestion across the rest of the shoulder, continue working from the phalangeal joint across both feet to the base of the big toes. All above conditions, with the cleansing diet, can be completely corrected for normal action in the shoulders.

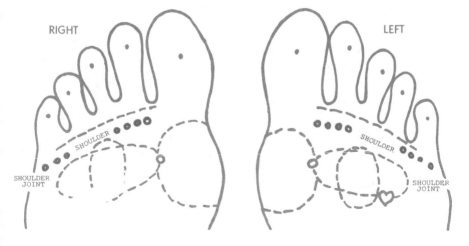

No. 31   Reflex points for shoulders

Painless Childbirth and Pelvic Reflexes
(No. 32)

All pelvic disorders respond rapidly to the reflex system. The same points are used for all of them. The following is a list of the main ones.

Prostate gland disorders
Piles and Hemorrhoids
Bladder troubles — all kinds
Menstral pains and cramps
Excessive or insufficient flow
Ovary and uterus troubles
Pressures, pains, congestion and tension during pregnancy
Some difficulties to becoming pregnant
Elimination of labor pains during childbirth

There is never a need for an operation on the **prostate gland.** So much pain and suffering can be avoided by following the cleansing diet and using Vita-Flex on all the pelvic control points. All swelling and congestion will be completely eliminated.

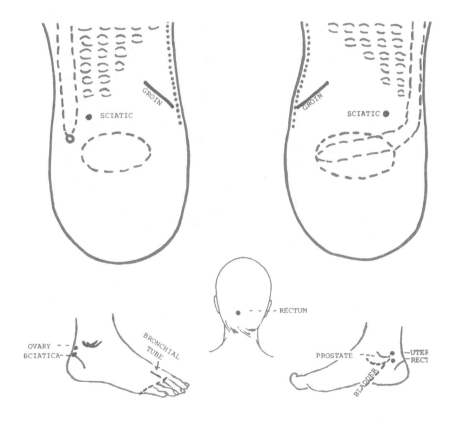

The Rectum Reflex Points

Rectum reflex points are on top of the achilles heel bone on both feet and the base of the skull, center back of head. These points for all conditions in the rectal area (such as piles and hemorrhoids) bring immediate relief. The **bladder** reflexes start at the rectal area and follow the heel bone down to the spine area and then to the **groin** area just beyond (No. 32). The **uterus** points are just above the rectal area. These points are also for the **testicles**. **Sciatica** is relieved by working on the points opposite to the rectal point on the outside of the heel. Other points are on the bottom of the feet near the heels and on outside of legs just below the knee (No. 35).

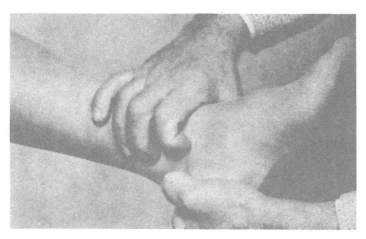

No. 33   Reflex points for prostate glands

Partial, and often complete, elimination of labor pains has been accomplished many times. Frequently the baby has been born in less than ten minutes from the first sign of activities. This has happened in the first birth as well as many births after. Many mothers have had many hours of labor with two or three other babies, but when Vita-Flex was properly used, the next birth was without pain and in minutes. The baby is a happier baby born without pain.

Pregnancy becomes more pleasant with no morning illnesses. Other bodily functions are made normal when proper food is eaten and Vita-

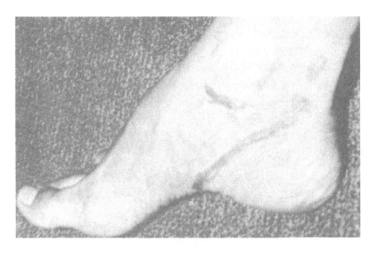

No. 34 Reflex points for prostate, bladder and groin

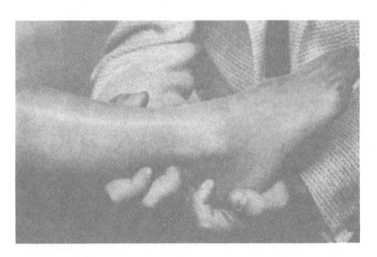

No. 35 Reflex points for sciatic and ovaries

Flex treatments are administered. All forms of animal and animal products must be abandoned. This includes honey, eggs, and dairy products.

During the last three months of pregnancy, about half of the diet should be our type of lemonade. This prevents a still birth in case the RH

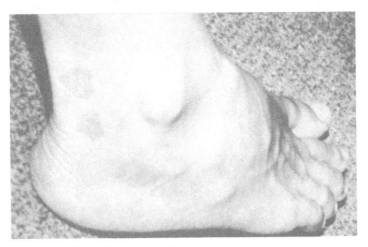

No. 36   Reflex points to sciatic and ovaries

factor exists in the mother. It also gives better nutrition for all other natural functions.

The shoulder adjustment for lengthening the leg is an important part for correcting the various pelvic organs — relieves menstral pains and lower back pains. This helps at the time of pregnancy.

The Taking of the Pill

The pill has many serious side effects. When man decides to manipulate the natural functions of the body, he pays a high price. Self control is always the best answer. Proper eating will produce normal activities in the body making for less stimulation and irritation of the sex glands.

There is no possible way to induce abortion with Vita-Flex. It is however, possible to prevent a miscarriage with these controls and proper diet. Sensible exercise is also beneficial.

Six Point Adjustment of Bones and Arches in Feet

In making correction of the arches and adjusting the bones many changes and improvements occur in other parts of the body. As the longitudinal arch is corrected curvatures in the spine are gradually made normal. As the metatarsal arch is corrected, lungs and thyroid conditions improve. In reality, the whole body responds and functions better as the feet are reshaped.

To make it possible to properly see the adjustments on paper we found it necessary to change feet from picture to picture. However, you do the complete 6 point adjustment on each foot without switching.

First adjustment:

The first position is to adjust the metatarsal arch. For the right foot the right thumb is pressed down on the small toe joint at right angles to the foot with the finger tips holding the upper part (toward the big toe) of the longitudinal arch for leverage (No. 37).

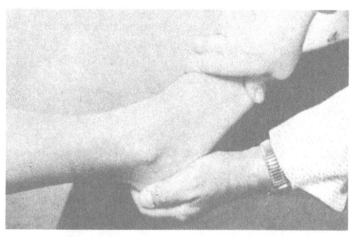

No. 37   First adjustment

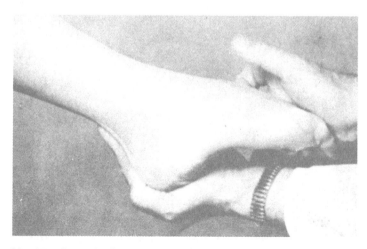

No. 38   Second adjustment

75

Second adjustment:

Retain the position of the first adjustment. Drop the palm of the right hand down over the toes, suspending the thumb and first finger with the big toe slightly showing (No. 38). Press all toes under and twist the foot from side to side in a half circle. This action loosens many parts of the foot as well as raising the metatarsal arch.

Third Adjustment (left foot)

Third adjustment using left hand holding the heel and the right grasping the foot firmly on top with the fingers wrapped around the bunion joint. Place the left elbow on the left knee. Twist the foot inward and under with the right hand while you press the center arch against the spine reflexes of the left hand. Move the thumb up and down the arch as you press on it. (No. 39).

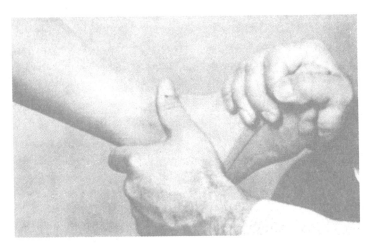

No. 39   Third adjustment

Fourth Adjustment (either foot)

Grasp the foot firmly with both hands just below the metatarsal pad. Press the toes down and the arch up and at the same time give several strong pulls with a shake. (No. 41)

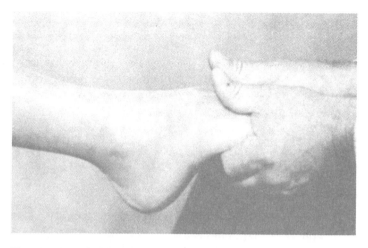

No. 40   Fourth adjustment

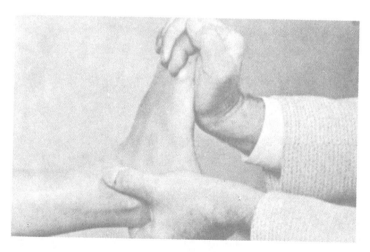

No. 41   Fifth adjustment

Fifth Adjustment (either foot)

Hold the heel with the left hand and place the base of the palm of the right hand against the metatarsal arch with the fingers curved over the toes. Push on the arch without jerking, several times and at the same time, pull the toes down. Straighten out the elbow as you push. This stretches the ligaments and tendons in the back of the legs. (No. 41).

77

Sixth adjustment:

Retain the position of the fifth adjustment and turn the foot several times in a large circle and then reverse. This helps to give relief to bunions. Further relief may be made by holding the big toe and forefinger with both hands (one on top of the other) and pulling quickly with several quick pulls.

The Hands
(No. 42)

There are as many reflexes on the hands as there are on the feet. Use them as a supplement to the feet reflexes. Also pains in the feet are relieved on the corresponding part of the hands. Under many conditions where it is difficult to use the feet, the reflexes in the hands work equally as well.

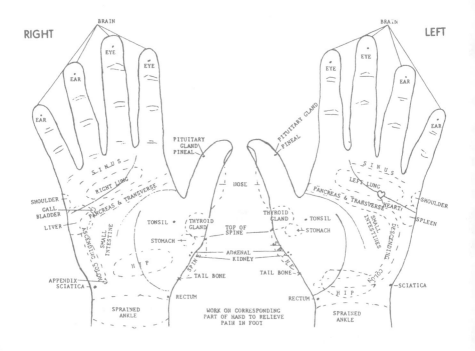

No. 42   **Reflex points on hands**

The Face

(No. 43)

The many reflexes on the face may be used from time to time as a supplement to the other points in the feet and hands. They are particularly useful when a complete body massage is given. A facial massage,

No. 43   Reflex points on face

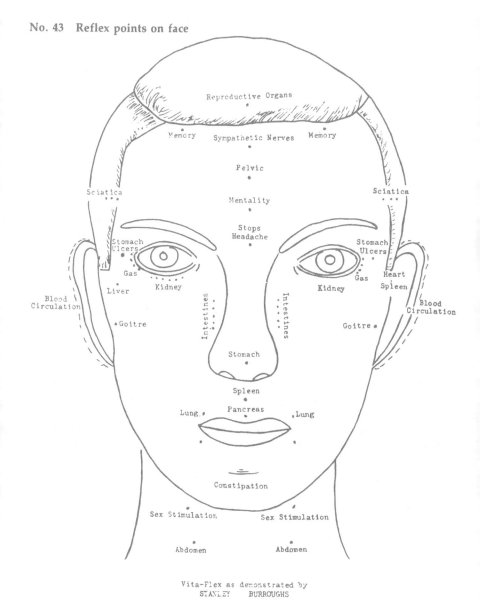

Vita-Flex as demonstrated by
STANLEY   BURROUGHS

while working on these reflex points, is very pleasant.

The few points that are used more often are the ones for the sciatic nerve, ovary, reproductive organs, and heart. Use them in connection with painless childbirth and pelvic disorders.

The other points are self explanatory. The same method, a pressure and a pull, is applied the same as on the feet and hands.

Reflexes in the Shoulder and Neck

The reflexes in the collar bone around the entire neck make corrections in all parts of the head directly above them. Either the fingers or the thumbs may be used for these control points. The correct way is to start on the inner side of the collar bone and roll the fingers around and under with firm medium pressure. Never hold these points — just press and release several times. (No. 44).

All of the foregoing are additional control points for relieving every kind of headache. Other points in the collar bone area relieve specific conditions of organs located in the head.

The eye reflexes are in the collar bone directly below the eyes. The ear reflexes are directly beneath the ears, further out on the collar bone. The same is true for fast relief of toothache, sore gums, other mouth problems, and the nose — this includes nose bleed and sinus problems. Just locate and work on the collar bone area directly beneath the affected part.

A form of neuritis in the face called a Tic causes extreme pain which is relieved immediately. Even drugs will not stop these pains. For sore, swollen, inflamed tonsils instant relief is felt. Tonsils should never be taken out. Work on the points below them around the collar bone.

For more relief of hearing problems, and specifically to increase hearing ability, there is a special form of ear treatment. Stand in back of the person. Place both index fingers, separately, into the ear openings as far as possible at the same time. With a pulling up and a side to side motion count a fast 20 as you massage firmly in the area. In the same opening, pull backward at the same time into both the ear openings, and proceed as follows:

Count a fast 20 as you pull up firmly with a side to side motion. (No. 45).

Count a fast 10 as you pull backward, with side to side motion. (No. 46).

Count a fast 10 as you pull downward, with side to side motion. (No. 47).

Now use the thumbs — push forward to a count of 10, with side to side motion. (No. 48).

Then give an extra pull upward. (No. 49).

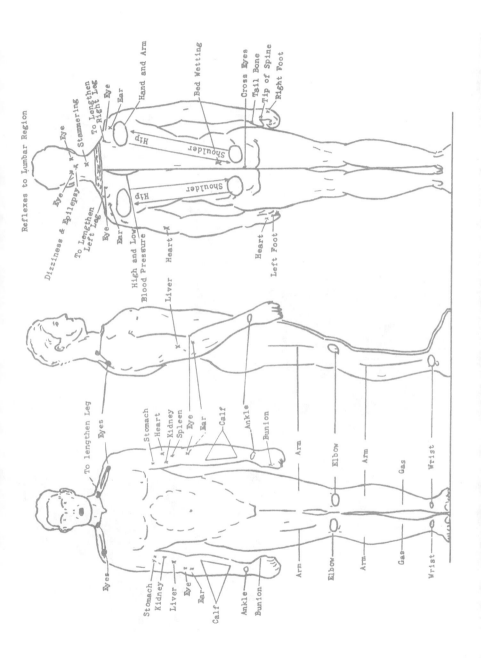

81

No. 45 Upward pull

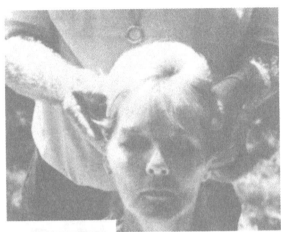

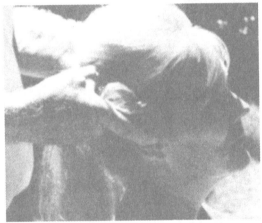

No. 46 Backward pull

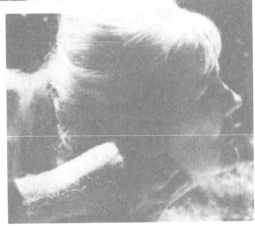

No. 47 Downward pull

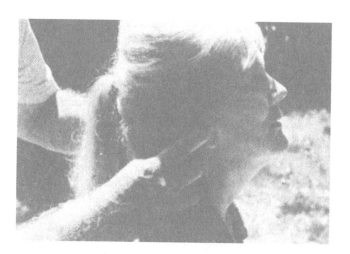

No. 48   Forward pull

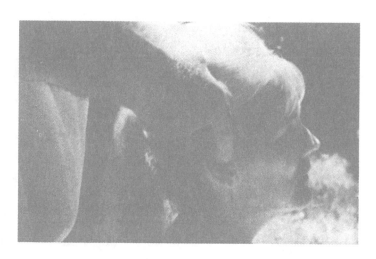

No. 49   Quick upward pull

Many people with earphones have been able to hear better without them and thus have no further need of them. This may be done as often as desired. The small organs of the inner ear are relieved of pressure and tension allowing them to function in normal, or near normal, fashion.

By working on the entire outer ear by pinching, circulation is increased over the entire body. There are many reflex points on the outer ear and at the entrance that produce good results all over the body. This is a quick way to warm up on a cold morning or at any time.

It should be noted that the same reflexes in the collar bone which relieve conditions in the head above also affect all parts of the body below in similar manner. The reflexes to the eyes are the same as to the stomach. The ear reflexes go to the liver, gall bladder and parts between and below. Use them to supplement the rest of the work.

One of the nicest parts of the Vita-Flex is that one is not limited to just one control point. There are many choices to make a complete correction.

Many of the reflex points go to other parts of the body other than the main point. A good example of this is found on the surface of the shoulder blades. (No. 50).

The best method to do the following work is to have the person sit on the floor in front of you — their back to you — while you sit in a chair.

The five dots near the top of the shoulder blades are control points for the thumbs and fingers. The two large inside points are the thumbs. The fingers extend outward from the thumbs.

These same points, plus the entire surface of the blades, control all parts of the hands, the wrists, the elbows and the arms.

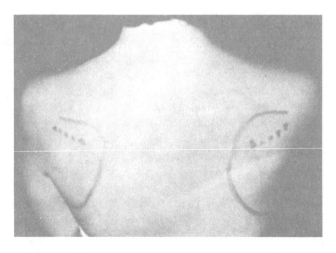

No. 50   Reflex points on shoulder blades

All the points on the shoulder blades also control the heart, lungs, and breasts on the left side and the lungs and breast on the right side. These same points also control and make corrections in the buttocks, the part you sit on.

Reflexes on the buttocks relieve and make corrections in the shoulder blades.

The reflex points in the entire length of the spine, on both sides, relieve and make corrections directly in front, directly through the body. The best way to do this is to "walk" with the thumbs up and down the sides of the spine. (No. 51).

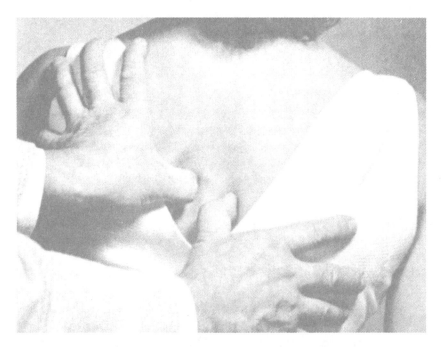

No. 51 Reflex points along entire length of the spine

Using the knees as fulcrum points over which to stretch and twist the back, pull the shoulders back and around with both hands. Use one knee at a time and then both knees. Place the knees in many places up and down the sides of the spine and across it. This exercise relaxes and loosens the spine and muscles for better movement and flexibility. (No.52).

To complete the procedure, moderately massage the shoulders, upper back and neck with a rolling and kneading action.

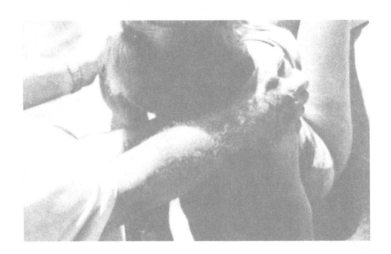

Katie's Wonderful Experience

Katie came to me a short time ago. For fourteen years she constantly suffered from pains in the tail bone and back. After much money and many systems of healing — her family was financially able to take her to the best specialists — her pain was still there. She was told she had to live with it. Whether sitting, lying, or walking there was no relief.

On her first visit Vita-Flex removed all pain from the back and tail bone. It never returned. She also had a large calcium spur on the tail bone which completely disappeared.

The third visit her badly prolapsed organs were raised and placed in correct position without the use of the scalpel or knife. They stayed where they belonged. One more visit and all conditions became normal. For the first time in years normal eliminations began and continued. The entire cost $30.00. No X-rays were needed. No examinations were made. Truly a perfect example of consistent and constant results with this finest in the healing arts.

The Head

There are as many reflexes on the head as there are on the feet and hands. I have not provided a complete chart of the head, but the control points follow the same pattern as those on feet, hands, and shoulder blades. The right and left points control the corresponding side of the body. The hair line in center front controls the atlas and the base of the center skull controls the tail bone. The rest of the spine is in between. Use the same type of pressure on the head as on the rest of the body.

Gently pulling the hair by running fingers through it and closing the fist tightly increases circulation in the scalp and growth of the hair. One of the nicest ways to induce sleep is pulling the hair and massaging the head.

Through extensive research and tests I discovered many important healing and corrective measures as actual structural changes were made by working on the head. Many spastic and palsy conditions were completely corrected by massaging and reshaping the head. (No. 53). The sutures in the head are always free to move to release pressures and tensions on the many part of the brain. Persons who were hopeless cases are now living a normal healthy life. I could cite many cases, but feel that a very special one should be described. This is not a rare case, but one of many which have been repeated over and over again, with this work. I will give the main highlights.

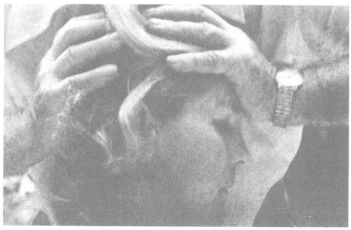

No. 53   **Reshape head**

Within the human computer there is stored complete data that is constantly on the alert to diagnose and prescribe what is needed and where it should go to correct the damage or supply the deficiency in any part or parts. The computer requires only the best cooperation of each individual to supply the raw materials designed by nature to fill the need.

The ability of the computer is strictly and completely automatic giving complete directions for every part to act in accordance with nature to serve unfalteringly to every need.

It is only when people ignore the simple natural needs of the body and become involved with drugs of any nature — legal or illegal — and a variety of denatured foods with excesses of any kind that people will become sick and crippled.

Even the computer will attempt to adjust and correct to the best of its ability with what is given it to work with.

All forms of illness reflect on the inability of its host to supply its needs rather than failure of the computer to perform to its desired perfection.

All the above completely eliminates the need for those outlandish expensive man made machines that man has built along with the costly errors of life and death of the humans involved.

With all this above knowledge of one's ability to diagnose, prescribe and heal all forms of diseases and illnesses, the wonder of it is that medicine should constantly be attempting to build ever more complicated and expensive machines at skyrocketing costs that can in no way compete or compare with the perfection of God's creation in every individual.

Remember — no man-made products, regardless of the cost, will every successfully replace the perfection of God's creations.

The high rising costs of man-made products have risen beyond the ability of man to survive any good it may tend to service such unnatural needs.

Medicine has reached a point where it has priced itself beyond the ability of man to buy its offerings.

Nature has kept its costs down to the normal level of supply and demand of simple fruits, herbs and other foods around the world.

Unscientific Medicine is always coming up with something new to prove it is a long way from meeting the needs of the people. But that something new always means something more expensive, more complicated, more dangerous, more prone to side effects and farther and farther away from simple natural methods that are far less expensive and far more effective.

After all, if they would but study nature more closely and learn what God has to offer, they might just find the answers — the simple answers that have been there all the time — that really works and simply works fast.

Nature can be and is the best teacher after all. Surely nature knows far more than any and all of the Medical Profession, because God ordained it, regardless of how close to the Divine they may think they are.

Were it not better we reverse our present destructive course and give nature a chance to show what God can do? Let us do it now. Nature has been around a lot longer than any of the Medical doctors or their systems and will still be there long after man made plans fade away.

Returning to natural methods can reduce the need for most of the hosptial care-less nursing care-less to no dangerous drugs and medication. Surgery can be almost a thing of the past, a horrible nightmare of faulty hopes of normal healing. Is this not what we need and are asking for? Just think of the misery and suffering and lives that can be saved by nature's methods. Are their lives not worth saving? Let nature prove its methods work successfully since present medical methods are fraught with a multitude of costly and deadly failures.

Medical Standards require nothing better — in spite of years of extensive and expensive research — than the practice of many addictive drugs and destructive surgery, until there is a cure. But if someone does come up with a cure for all diseases they will be treated — prosecuted — as a common criminal as treating is more lucrative than a cure.

The Amazing Story of Rose

I owned a health club in Honolulu on Keeaumoku Street at the time. One morning in 1970, a girl of about 29 years hobbled in to talk with me. She was severely spastic from birth. Her speech was difficult and halting. Her mouth was badly twisted and her fingers could not open. She walked sideways with a bad twist. She was the worst spastic I have ever seen who was still able to be on her feet. I have seen many like her, but none quite so bad.

She sat down and we talked,. Her name was Rose. Many of her friends and acquaintances called her "Crooked Rose". During her lifetime many medical and various systems had failed to make any change in her condition. To them she was hopeless. She must live with it.

After telling me this history of her life, she then asked "Can you help me"? Of course I could. I knew with God's help and the unlimited healing power behind the entire work at my command, she would not be let down.

She came daily, week after week, hitch-hiking from the North Shore. Often she walked many blocks both directions with great difficulty. The important thing is — she came.

And little by little changes came too. Nothing drastic; just a steady response. After about three months she walked in with a present for me. She had made me a very nice shirt with hands that were almost useless before. She was now talking freely and walking almost straight.

Seven months of treatments and a very pretty girl began a new life as a normal being. Later she married and had a normal child. Her friends couln't believe that this was "Crooked Rose".

Shouldn't a system such as this receive the highest acclaim and respect? And the work be made available to the entire world?

The cause of Rose's condition — doctors at delivery had used instruments to pull the baby by the head causing pressure on the brain and nerves inside. The correction was made by Vita-Flex structural changes, correct diet and color therapy.

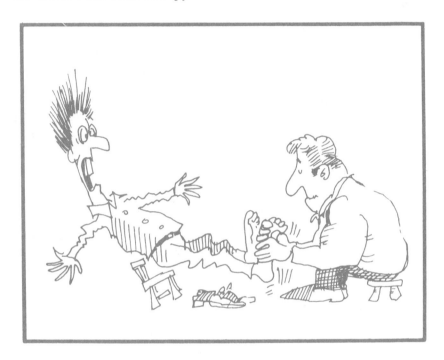

The Full Vita-Flex Treatment

Since all parts of the body work in harmony with each other, a full reflex massage is the most desirable way to stimulate, activate, and relax the entire body.

When the treatment is completed a tingling sensation with lightness and flexability permeates the entire body.

Tensions, pains, stiffness and that over-all feeling of tiredness disappear as complete relaxation replaces them. At the same time one can be extremely active in various ways or let go and peacefully lie down and relax. Sleep comes at night quickly and gently so as never to require any form of sleeping pills or potions.

The entire procedure may be done daily for no harm can ever be done at any time.

The approximate order to give a full treatment is as follows: (Refer to the charts to locate the reflex points and apply pressure as described and illustrated on the preceding pages.)

    1. Right foot:

appendix
ascending colon
liver and gall bladder
transverse colon and pancreas

2. Left foot: (continuing across)
   transverse colon and pancreas
   spleen
   descending colon and across to tail bone
   tail bone
   up spine to top of spine
   kidneys and adrenal gland
   stomach
   thyroid and parathyroid gland on bunion joint
   bronchial on top of foot
   tonsil on bottom
   nose — inside and outside of big toe
   back of head and neck
   pituitary and pineal gland
   sinus — reach over toes
   lungs — reach over toes
   shoulder
   heart (on left only)

3. Right foot: (again)
   tail bone
   up spine to top of spine
   kidney and adrenal glands
   stomach
   thyroid and parathyroid gland on bunion joint
   thyroid and parathyroid on bunion joint
   bronchial on top of foot
   tonsil on bottom of foot
   nose — inside and outside of big toe
   back of head and neck
   pituitary and pineal gland
   sinus — reach over toes
   lungs — reach over toes
   shoulder

4. Right foot (continued) — Lower pelvic area and painless
   childbirth:
   prostate
   rectum
   bladder and groin
   uterus
   sciatic nerve
   ovary

sciatic on bottom of foot
sciatic in the leg
5. Left foot lower pelvic area — also painless childbirth:
    prostate
    rectum
    bladder and groin
    uterus
    sciatic nerve
    ovary
    sciatic on bottom of foot
    sciatic in the leg
6. Six point adjustment start with right foot
7. Special troubles — go over any spots that were found sore or
    where person has troubles
8. Shin bone
9. Hands all over — every spot as a supplement to feet
    (also takes pains out of foot from the treatment.)
    stretch hand
10. Ear and eye reflex in elbow — both arms
    Heart (Left side only) hand and arm (first one then the other — a
    pumping motion.)
11. Seated on floor, back to operator
    work across shoulders for constipation and lower back troubles
    lengthen legs
    eyes and ears
    thumb-walk up and down spine
    all over blade of shoulder for hands, hips and breast
    work all around inside of collar bone
    press knee at various points in back and stretch
12. Ears
    up to count of 20
    back 10
    down 10
    forward 10
    quick lift up
13. Reflex at back of head for eyes, headaches and rectum
14. Head
    press to shoulder — left then right
    twist to stretch (gently left then right)
    arm behind head — press head one way and the arm the
    opposite to stretch
    reflexes all over head, press head to shape
    squeeze hair
15. Face
    heart on left

ovaries and sciatic on both sides
(use other reflexes on face if condition requires)

General Procedure for Full Body Massage

Massage with medium deep, long strokes where possible. This is only a condensed version. Class work and experience is necessary for a complete work.

Before starting massage put a small amount of coconut oil on subject and then use massage and skin conditioner. The recipe is found on page 100 in the Special Hints.

Subject lies on back

1. Each foot separately (use both hands)
2. Each leg and foot
3. Both legs and hips at same time using long strokes
4. Quick kneading of legs
5. Stomach
6. Chest and shoulders
7. Each hand-arm-shoulder (arm across chest then arm behind head)
8. Facial, neck, turn head side to side, pull head back
9. Both arms over head; long strokes, tug-twist

Subject lies on stomach

1. Each foot and calf (knee bent perpendicular) bring heel to buttock
2. Bottoms of each foot using both thumbs — downward tug
3. Each leg separately (concentrate on inner thighs for women)
4. Both legs at the same time
5. Quick kneading of legs
6. Kneading buttocks
7. Back; long strokes — one hand on the other, thumb-knuckle along spine, hands in a swimming motion, (cover back with towel) hands crisscrossed over spine (subject inhales deeply first, repeat with head turned to other side, then up on elbows)
8. Cover with towel, quick kneading of back and legs
9. Rapping with fists, slapping (use vibrator if available)

The Foot Roller

Often when the need for a good treatment arises there is no one around to help. To meet this need a most effective foot exerciser for the reflexes in the feet, hands, and other parts has been designed by the author. (No. 54).

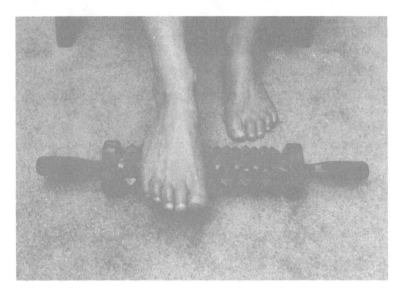

No. 54   The foot roller

The device is a special type of roller with staggered, fine-pointed pegs, placed close enough together so as not to dig in too deeply with heavy pressure. They are far enough apart to reach all points as one rolls both feet back and forth. The socks may be left on for a more comfortable and relaxing feeling. In just a few minutes tensions, drowsiness, weariness, and pain disappear. The entire body responds to the stimulation for a more active life. Tense and tired feet get fast relief.

It may be used on the back by another person to great advantage — it feels very good and relaxing. Use a towel or other material between the roller and the back to soften the pressure.

It is especially useful and effective on bulging spots that need reducing. Use a towel for these conditions also.

The foot roller duplicates the effect of walking barefoot over rough and stony ground. It may be used as often as desired with no ill effect.

The foot roller may be obtained direct from the publisher.

The Use of a Vibrator

For a number of years I have been using a very heavy vibrator on the feet, back and other parts of the body. This is done at the end of the foot treatment and at the end of the body massage. It is an excellent method of completing the full treatment. The tingling and lightness experienced by the body is a superb finish to a most pleasant total experience.

94

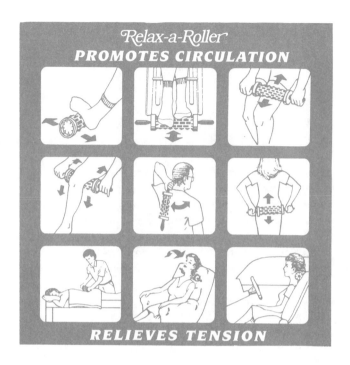

Relax-a-Roller

PROMOTES CIRCULATION

RELIEVES TENSION

The Relax-a-Roller is a foot and body massager designed to create a reflex or pressure point massage similar to Vita-Flex or Reflexology. It is recommended by Chiropractors, Naturopaths and Reflexologists.

The Relax-a-Roller can be ordered through Burroughs Books for $20.00 per unit plus $4.00 for shipping. CA Residents please add 7.25% tax.

Send to: **Burroughs Books
3702 S. Virginia St.
Ste. # G-12 Box 346
Reno, NV 89502-6030**

Dealer inquiries invited.

**Manufactured by Vita-Gem Enterprises
Victoria, B.C. Canada**

CHAPTER III:

Yoga

Because the ancient arts of Vita-Flex, color therapy, and yoga are so closely related in their actions on the body, I felt compelled to include a word about yoga. But since I am only a beginning layman as far as yoga is concerned, I felt it necessary to call upon an expert for help.

While we do not consider yoga as a form of religion in any sense of the word, we do consider the natural laws and benefits of the use of yoga to be of the utmost importance in building and retaining more complete and balanced health, poise and suppleness of the physical body. Since the physical body is a part of trinity of being then as the body strives toward perfection then our mind and spirit also receives great benefits from its accomplishments.

The practice of yoga allows our mind and spirit to function more freely and perfectly since it is not held back for a sick and ailing weakly body.

I consider it a privilege to present this work taken directly from the original and authentic Sanskrit so that you, the reader, may know how important this activity and practice became to an ancient people.

Sometimes, and generally speaking, original works from the past have not always been enough and sufficient for all the millions of people who live in the years that follow so they have altered or improved them to suit themselves. This can be considered as progress and to these people they have found a more complete answer or just another way.

It is not my purpose to justify or condemn any or all of these practices. I do suggest that you search out and choose only the very best to suit your purpose.

In my own experiences I have found that as we develop a more perfect body and better understanding of how it works with the mind and spirit, we no longer need to spend many hours of medative inactivity to accomplish and achieve higher spiritual development or create harmony with all phases of the trinity.

I, as many others have found that it is also very beneficial, if not necessary, to train the muscles and mind to many of the more speedy and active forms of exercise. These activities train the mind, muscles and nerves to perform alertly and quickly to possible emergencies which constantly occur in our modern civilization. This creates a natural balance of both the slow and the fast type of exercise.

By using the Vita-Flex, color therapy and the best of balanced nutrition with balanced exercise we have taken nothing away from the original findings of the ancients but have added great and wonderful benefits to their experiences.

Since Vita-Flex and color therapy are also a great healing knowledge discovered and used successfully by the ancients we feel highly indebted to them for their discoveries and use. We feel that with all this great knowledge properly put to use as a completeness we no longer need to waste our time with needless hours of long concentrated meditation. Often we find that short periods — minutes — of decentration and relaxation we can achieve the equal or better results than many long periods of meditation.

As you, or if you do go through the experiences of yoga, consider the above facts and utilize only the very best of teachers as your instructor. The right one for you may be hard to find so in the mean time make use of what is available and keep searching.

William C. Finley has generously offered this chapter on yoga taken directly from the original Sanskrit. I present it knowing that it can add greatly to your life.

Haṭha Yoga

Haṭha Yoga, one of the many recently popular branches of Yoga, is the practice or exercise of various static physical postures of the body called āsanas, and breath control called prāṇāyāma. The āsanas and prāṇāyāma are two of the eight parts described in the aṣṭāṅga, or eight-limbed Yoga, originally written in the oldest known foundational text on Yoga called the **Yoga Sūtras of Patañjali.** Thousands of years ago in India, a man known traditionally as Patañjali taught a scientific eight step method of physical, emotional, mental and spiritual culture to enable the soul of man to free itself from his psycho-physical covering to attain its pristine purity and reunite with God. Patañjali enumerated in Saṁskṛta in Sūtra II (29): "Yama, niyama, āsana, prāṇāyāma, pratyāhāra, dhāraṇā, dhyāna, and samādhi are the eight limbs."

There are five yamas or rules of self-control:

1. Ahiṁsā — Non-violence in thought, word, and deed against any living being
2. Satya — Truthfulness
3. Asteya — Non-stealing
4. Brahmacarya — Continence
5. Aparigraha — Non-possessiveness, detachment

And, there are five niyamas or observances to cultivate positive virtues:
1. Śauca — Purity in body, emotions, and mind
2. Saṁtoṣa — Contentment, equanimity, and tranquility
3. Tapas — Austerity, will power, and self-discipline
4. Svādhyāya — Self-study of scriptures and philosophy
5. Īśvarapraṇidhāna — Submission to the will of God

These ten rules and observances are the moral precepts and ethical foundation to be studied, learned, and followed by a yogin in order to slowly and methodically withdraw the attention from emotional and mental turmoil and disturbances in the world to create a calm internal environment in preparation for later meditation.

In the third step Patañjali prescribed a series of psycho-physical āsanas to prepare the body and mind for long periods of meditation. The second standard treatise on Yoga named the **Hathapradīpikā of Svātmārāma** gave only 15 classical āsanas to perform, rather than the legendary 84. Svātmārāma said in Sūtra I (17): "Āsanas give steadiness, health, and lightness."

The fourth limb of prāṇāyāma, control and regulation of inspiration, retention, and expiration of breath, was done by a student only under the guidance of a fully competent teacher after many years of performing āsanas successfully and adherence to a strict diet which excluded meat, fish, fowl, and eggs. This further purifies the mind and prepares the body for meditation.

After these four preliminary phases of moral cultivation and physical culture which help eliminate the external causes of distraction, the mind becomes fit for concentration exercises.

Part five called pratyāhāra is the conscious removal or withdrawal of the attention by the mind from the senses and its objects.

Dhāraṇā is concentration, the fixing or holding of the attention to one place or object.

Dhyāna is contemplation, intense concentration in an unbroken flow of attention at that place or on that object.

Samādhi, the eighth and final step, is the state of intense contemplation where the attention is merged or united with that place or object only, and is not aware of itself. It is an extraordinary state of complete absorption where consciousness is unhampered by mental fluctuations.

Samyama, the simultaneous practice of dhāraṇā, dhyāna, and samādhi, produces in stages light, power, knowledge, and higher consciousness or vibration.

Patañjali described nine varieties of mental samādhi, which culminated finally in a systematic withdrawal of the attention from the physical realm and enabled the yogin to concentrate his attention within at will. This is the real and true definition and objective of Patañjali's eight step Yoga system. He said in the famous Sūtra I (2): "Yoga is the control of the waves of the mind." The entire purpose of the original eight limbs of Patañjali was to directly or indirectly control the mind through continuous self-control and discipline. The yogin then remained within the natural laws of physical; emotional, and mental health, which automatically created a more calm inner environment, raised his vibration level, and prepared him for meditation. In all eight phases a competent living teacher was assumed to be necessary. After this, the yogin began the initial stages of higher spiritual meditation. At this point the teachings of the **Yoga Sūtra** stop and the yogin received the technique of spiritual meditation (which always remained unwritten) from the living guru of his time. He was taught how to vacate the body at will to begin the spiritual journey to higher planes.

Gradually, throughout the centuries after Patañjali's original work on Yoga, many fragmentary Yoga systems came into vogue. Today we see a dizzying variety of practices such as laya yoga, karma yoga, śakti yoga, kuṇḍdalinī yoga, mantra yoga, bhakti yoga, yantra yoga, dhyāna yoga, rāja yoga, jñāna yoga, samādhi yoga, etc. Certain personalities or schools concentrated on and emphasized more just one limb or part of the original eight-fold path to the exclusion or neglect of the other parts. And so, much of the real practice of Yoga has been lost, and a student must search hard and long to find that rare, competent Yoga teacher or living adept.

For the purposes of this volume we are concerned mainly with the psycho-physical āsanas and diet of Haṭha Yoga. They have a parallel healthy effect on the body. Like the purifying diet and Vita Flex, the yogic diet and exercises undertaken even for a short time promotes health, cleansing, and a higher vibration.

The psycho-physical āsanas affect both body and mind, and are generally classified.into meditative and cultural exercises. Originally, the meditative āsanas such as the well-known cross-legged lotus varieties and kneeling postures, were static poses used only for long periods of meditation. Only much later in medieval times were cultural āsanas developed as aids to tone up the body and help to hold the meditative postures longer in those who had weaker bodies. The cultural āsanas helped create a psycho-physical condition conducive to better health and performance of meditative poses. As hundreds of years passed, these unique Yoga gymnastic exercises became systematized and were mistaken for Yoga itself. Instead of being known for their true function of making the body stronger so that the yogin could meditate longer, the āsanas became an end in themselves and the real Yoga practice of mind control and advancement to spiritual meditation was undermined, distorted, and then forgotten.

Later, however, it became apparent that the cultural āsanas had a very good influence on health, having a healing and corrective effect on a variety of ailments and disorders in the body. The cultural āsanas were found to promote relaxation, remove fatigue, loosen tight joints, improve circulation and assimilation, dissipate stress and tension, increase spinal flexibility, stimulate the nervous system, increase the energy flow in the physical and subtle bodies, dissolve subtle energy blocks, build and tone the entire muscle structure, especially in the spinal area, for better posture and balance, massage pelvic viscera, and increase concentration by putting one in conscious contact with your nervous system.

A brief routine of twenty minutes a day, especially for people having too little exercise in sedentary occupation in offices and cities, is enough to accomplish all these benefits. The following nine āsanas should be done smoothly, slowly, and in a steady manner without jerks. Done with regularity and perseverance, they will furnish this minimal yogic routine, The cultural āsanas are more static exercises, rather than dynamic or fast Western calisthenics. The nature of the yogic exercise is different because it acts on nerves more than muscles. The postures should always be stable and comfortable. There should never be any undue strain, tension, or pain in their practice. Gradually and progressively, these slow, controlled stretching postures should be learned only under the guidance of a good Haṭha Yoga teacher. There are many ways to do āsanas incorrectly, and their benefits can be increased fivefold by having a good teacher.

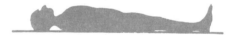

I. Śavāsana — corpse pose: "Lying supine on the ground like a corpse is śavāsana. It wards off fatigue and brings mental relaxation." (H.P. I — 32) Lying prone in a state of relaxed awareness or controlled alertness is the most important exercise in Haṭha Yoga. It is simple to understand, but difficult to do. Willful and conscious relaxation is very hard to accomplish, but very important in our tension and stress filled world of today. Śavāsana correctly done is excellent for everyone, especially heart patients and those with psychosomatic disorders.

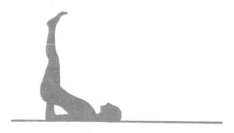

II. Viparīta karanī — topsy turvy pose: This is a modified shoulder stand with feet in the air and the sacral area supported by the hands. This inverted pose should be done progressively and increased slowly day by day. "It can only be learned by the instructions of a teacher." (H.P. III — 78, 80) The topsy turvy pose is good for circulation and visceraptosis, displacement and dysfunction of pelvic and abdominal organs.

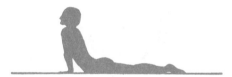

III. Halāsana — plough pose: This is a forward bending pose which is a systematic spinal stretch done while starting from a prone position. The plough should also be done cautiously in stages under supervision. Halāsana facilitates full spinal flexibility from the sacrum to the cervical vertebrae.

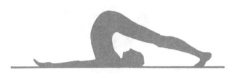

IV. Bhujamgāsana — cobra pose: The cobra is a backward bend of the spine from the hips to the head. It is helpful for building back muscles along the spine and toning up the viscera.

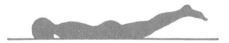

V. Śalabhāsana — locust pose: This complements the cobra pose as it is another posterior bend from the hips to the feet. The locust strengthens the lower lumbar region and leg muscles. This helps prevent and relieve lower back pains and aches.

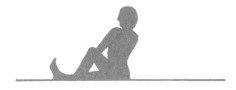

VI. Vakrāsana — twisted pose: This is a gentle twisting of the spine

101

in a sitting position. This spinal twist is helpful for loosening, lengthening, and stretching muscles and ligaments in the spinal column to keep the entire spine flexible and free from fixations.

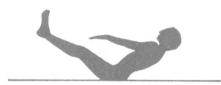

VII. Naukāsana — boat pose: While sitting, the legs and trunk are raised about 30 degrees off the ground with the arms parallel to the floor. The boat posture is good for toning up and slimming the entire abdominal area.

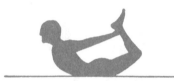

VIII. Dhanurāsana — bow pose: The bow pose is a complete backward bend, the result of combining the cobra and the locust poses, performed on the stomach while holding the ankles. It is excellent for the building and toning of back muscles, abdominal massage, assimilation, and overweight conditions.

IX. Paścimatānāsana — posterior stretching pose: This is a relaxed forward bend while sitting and holding the legs or feet as far forward as possible. This forward bend strengthens back muscles and the lumbar region. It is good for relieving sciatica, stimulating abdominal organs, and removing excess fat from the stomach and hips.

There are many other āsanas and their variations, but these basic nine exercises put the spine through its entire range of natural movement to affect the whole body. For best results this order of performing the āsanas should be followed. Also, all yogic routines should begin with 1 minute or more of śavāsana, followed by another minute of śavāsana after each and every pose, and ended with five minutes of śavāsana.

Thus we have given a brief description and the benefits of a minimal yogic exercise program to be learned from a good teacher, which should suffice to assist any serious student towards steadiness, lightness, and good health.

CHAPTER IV:

Special Needs and Problems

Special Hints

The following hints encompass some of the best of the simple and natural aids which are of great benefit in the correction of various minor inconveniences that may develop at any time in our lives.

Oil of Clove

Oil of clove is invaluable for many things. It is especially good for skin cancers, warts, and corns. With the finger, apply a small amount on warts or corns. Wait a short time. With an emery stick, scrape the top off and apply oil again. Repeat this several times daily until wart or corn disappears. Do the same thing for skin cancer. These forms of blemishes are not caused by a virus, but are a form of fungus growth feeding on acid elimination in the skin. (Our type of diet, incidentally, prevent these conditions from forming in the beginning.)

Clove oil stops the pain in the following conditions:

Use a small amount on the gums for toothache, and swollen or sore parts of the mouth. Use for canker sores.

Use for all insect stings and bites (wasp and mosquito, for example), scratches, small burns, and sores that are slow in healing. It is an excellent disinfectant. It takes the sting out of nettles and poison oak.

Use your finger to put a small amount on the back of the tongue for sore throat or a tickling cough.

For those who wish to quit smoking — every time you have the desire for a smoke place — with your finger — a small amount on the tongue and you immediately lose your desire to smoke. This is the easy way if you really want to quit.

Bay Rum

Bay Rum makes a nice after shave lotion. The benefits received from Bay Rum are many. For infections, irritations, and itching inside the ear dip a Q-tip in the solution and place inside the ear for immediate relief. Use as often as needed with no side effects.

For dandruff and itchy scalp — use straight and rub into the scalp.

For all irritations on the skin surfaces it is very healing. It brings fast relief to irritated parts in the groin.

Use as an astringent for the face and neck — very refreshing. Also helps to relieve sunburn and chapped skin.

Camphor and Camphor Cubes

When taking a bath in a tub, place 2 camphor cubes in the water. It is an excellent skin softener and relieves itching.

Camphor liniment is excellent for tired and sore muscles. It is a super skin conditioner. It relieves itching and pain of insect bites.

Camphor makes an excellent inhalent. It clears the head.

Castor Oil

Castor oil is fine for corns, warts, and other skin blemishes.

Coconut Oil

Coconut is one of the finest oils for the skin. It softens, removes wrinkles, and adds body to the skin. It helps to prevent sunburn and windburn. It is a fine dressing for the hair.

Honey

While honey does more harm than good internally (see page 12), it is especially good for many conditions externally. It heals many kinds of sores. It is very good for infections and in poultices.

Osage Rub

Osage Rub is an excellent commercial product for tired and sore muscles and skin. It is very cooling and refreshing. It makes an ideal after shave lotion. On a warm day, rub a small amount on the face and neck as a cooling agent.

Peppermint Oil

Peppermint oil is excellent for headaches. It clears the sinus. It cools and refreshes to enable free breathing. Place a small amount on one hand (tip the bottle upside down with the palm tight against the opening). Rub the two palms together and then inhale through the nose and mouth for a short time. Later, place the palms on forehead and back of the head. It is very cooling — especially helpful in case of fevers. A small amount of peppermint on the finger and rubbed inside the mouth makes the mouth feel refreshed and cool.

Wintergreen

The true oil of Wintergreen is superior to the synthetic, so use it if possible. The synthetic will work, but not as well.

It relieves pain in warts and corns. It is an excellent product for sore and painful muscles and joints. It is very warming — increases circulation.

Witch Hazel

Witch Hazel is an excellent astringent and skin conditioner. It is a natural for an after shave application. It gives fast relief for sore and irritated skin all over the body.

Vinegar

Pure Apple Cider Vinegar is a simple and safe, natural antibiotic. It may be used on the outside or inside of the body. If used on the outside, full strength is completely safe. If used on the inside, it must be diluted.

Athletes Foot: Four to five days of frequent use on feet will clear the condition. Use it periodically from then on to prevent a return. Works faster than other medication.

Chapped Sore Hands: Any fungus condition on hands or other parts of the body, is quickly corrected with straight vinegar.

Dandruff: Straight vinegar on the head clears dandruff very quickly.

Ring Worm: (on any part of the body): Vinegar often does the job of stopping it. Often stronger methods are necessary. For these occasions, pure peppermint oil works well. If this is not available, a commercial product called "Heet" works very well. The more frequently these products are applied, the faster the condition disappears.

Sore Throat: Vinegar and water — half and half — is an excellent gargle for sore throat and to cut mucus. It is also excellent for canker sores and infections or swellings in the mouth.

Indigestion or Gas: 2 teaspoons of vinegar in a glass of water; may be consumed with the meal or any time afterwards as needed. Use the same amount to stop dysentary or diarrhea — take it every hour until the condition has cleared. However, diarrhea can be very helpful for cleaning and eliminating of surplus toxins from the body. Do not be in too big a rush to stop the body's natural process in the cleansing.

Household uses: A vinegar application will loosen a rusted or corroded bolt.

For clearing stopped up sink pour ½ cup of baking soda down the drain. Add ½ glass of vinegar and cover for a minute.

Two tablespoons of vinegar and 2 tablespoons of maple syrup to a quart of water will aid in keeping cut flowers longer.

½ cup of ammonia and 3 tablespoons of vinegar added to each quart of warm water is excellent for washing windows without leaving film or streaks.

Massage and Skin Conditioner

All of the different oils and solutions may be added together to make one of the finest massage solutions available. Each ingredient complements and aids the other to do a remarkable job for most above conditions.

Into a gallon container add:
1 pt. Bay Rum
1 pt. Witch Hazel
3 oz. Osage Rub
2 tbsp. Camphor liniment
1 tbsp. Oil of Clove
¼ oz. Peppermint Oil
¼ oz. Wintergreen Oil
1 oz. Castor Oil
2 oz. Heet (a commercial product)
4 oz. Good hand and body cream
3 pt. Rubbing Alcohol
1 oz. Apple Cider Vinegar
1 oz. Eucalyptus
2 pt. Water
2 oz. Honey (optional)

Mix all together and use straight at any time for a most beneficial and refreshing tonic for the face and skin. These ingredients may be found in a drug store or barber supply.

The Abuse of Drugs

To descend to the bottom of the pit is the hard way to find that this is not the path to the heavenly bliss that one may have heard so much about. Many young people have sincerely sought "instant samadhi" through drugs, only to discover too late it was an abortive route. The many "drug abuse clinics" and "rehabilitation centers", engage in piecing together the shattered and fragmented lives of our youth, are a symbol of our age.

The need for drugs of any kind has been greatly exaggerated. The over-development, manufacture, and sale of these drugs has systematically created a world of unnecessary addiction. The freedom with which these drugs are used staggers the imagination.

For the most part use of drugs has been minimal throughout history. It took modern chemistry, medicine, and greed, for profits and power to create a monster of addiction and suffering. The drugs that were used to relieve suffering created misery and suffering by addiction.

Not wanting to be left out, the younger generation has understandably taken everything and anything they could get their little fingers into and made a big thing of it. Having no more common sense or control than adults, much damage to their bodies and minds has resulted. Crime, loss of property and life, has steadily increased with the increase in the use of these drugs.

Getting even, or striking back at our parents and the adult world in general, for their imperfections and lack of understanding is the hard way to prove a point. It only adds more problems to both parties involved. Must one become involved in the weaknesses and depravity of adult civilization in the entirely justifiable search for freedom?

The price we pay for this abuse has reached and gone beyond our ability to pay for and live with it. The trend must be reversed. The development, growth, and manufacture of these useless addictives must be eliminated from our society, if we ever hope to produce a better world to live in. Only when we create it can we ever hope to live in a better world.

Any possible good that drugs have to offer can easily be duplicated and improved upon by simple and natural methods. If these drugs were not manufactured and distributed by unscrupulous people in the adult world, there would be no possible way our children could procure them.

It is time for the younger generation to completely review the whole situation. It is the duty of the young and the vital to bring about the needed changes in our society. Why wait for the next generation? This creative renewal cannot be accomplished by wallowing in the filth the older generations have created. Don't let someone's greed for money and power be your downfall.

Drugs do not bring one closer to the Divine or free one from those imaginary shackles. As the effect of the drugs wear off, the old problems are still unsolved and new ones have been added. Drugs separate the psychic body from the physical. It is most difficult for the soul to remain healthy while the body is sick with drugs. While the psychic body is out of the physical, many adverse conditions can occur. Protective controls are gone, leaving the body wide open to destructive forces or lower spirit entities.

Leaving the body under such adverse conditions brings our psychic into an imaginary world of illusion or to the bottom of the pit of utter confusion. Any point there, or in between, can destroy the physical and leave us stranded in the world of confusion which only delays our journey to the higher realms of being. Heaven, God, or the finer things in life are not found in the doping and supressing of the physical body.

The drug way is surely the hard way to find reality. Keeping the mind and body free from the degrading effect of drugs gives it a strong incentive to advance more rapidly to the most desired form of living.

CHAPTER V:

The Miracle of Light and Color

The history of healing with color is very extensive and most impressive. The results of color use are so convincing, that one must eventually conclude that all healings begins and ends with color.

Records taken from the pyramids reveal the use of colors in healing among the ancient Egyptians. Their system appears to have been highly advanced and to have given excellent results.

The Rosicrucian society with its highly developed knowledge of esoteric teachings, has used color healing successfully since the 15th century.

In the latter part of the 19th century, Dr. Edwin D. Babbitt wrote **The Principles of Light and Color.** His work, the first major contribution in modern times, told of the many values in color healing nearly a century ago.

In the early part of the 20th century, Colonel Dinshah Pshadi Ghadali developed color healing to an exceptionally high degree.

In spite of the extensive development and successful use of color in healing, the orthodox medical authorities have consistently denied its worth and persecuted those who chose to use and spread the available knowledge about it. The rapid spread of color therapy around the world continues, however, in spite of all attempts to stop it. The truth will not be denied.

The writings of Edgar Cayce provide additional evidence that color has many healing qualities.

Without further enumerating authors and titles, we may point out that some two dozen significant works on color therapy, within the current century, abundantly demonstrate that there is far more to color than just something pretty to look at.

The many writings, results, and conclusions are so impressive as to warrant an all-out effort of further research into this highly effective system of healing. Indeed, extensive research and experience over many years with actual cases of every variety has already advanced color therapy to a high peak of efficiency and simplicity. All during the time of its development results have constantly proven that color is superior in every way to any form of medication, shots, chemotherapy, or surgery — and with absolutely no adverse side effects.

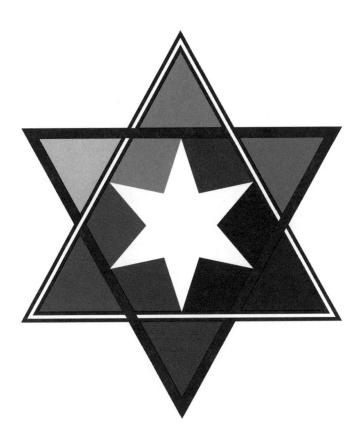

Wave Length of Various Colors

Red
  1/37,000″ or 6865 Å or 436.7*
Orange
  1/40,125″ or 6330 Å or 473.6*
Yellow
  1/43,250″ or 5873 Å or 510.5*
Lemon
  1/46,375″ or 5477 Å or 547.4*
Green
  1/49,500″ or 5131 Å or 584.3*
Turquois
  1/52,625″ or 4827 Å or 621.2*

Blue
  1/55,750″ or 4556 Å or 658.0*
Indigo
  1/58,875″ or 4314 Å or 694.9*
Violet
  1/62,000″ or 4097 Å or 731.8*
Purple
  1/52,625″ or 4827 Å or 621.2*
Magenta
  1/49,500″ or 5131 Å or 584.3*
Scarlet
  1/46,375″ or 5477 Å or 547.4*

* Stands for trillions (or million millions) of vibrations per second
Å Stands for angstrom units – a scientific unit of measurement: 1Å = 1/254,000,000″

The continued superior results in untold thousands of patients and students around the world are such that people can no longer be denied the right to use color for healing. This work should be highly promoted and taught so that more people may have the great advantages it has to offer.

Einstein writes that all forms of matter are light waves in motion. All colors represent the energy of light waves in motion vibrating at distinct and measurable rates.

All created things have colors, tones, and forms of their own. Every created color tone, and thought associated with it, becomes a living thing to torture man or exalt him according to his use or abuse of the natural laws. Colors are vibrations of creation. Color is the result of chemical action. Color creates chemical action and matter.

Whether their practitioners are aware of it or not, all systems of healing depend on color, and the chemical action in the body which produces color, to bring about any kind of change in body functions. Even in medication a variety of colors is ever present. The chemicals of which these medicines are composed contain mineral oxides and compounds. When medication is taken into the body and utilized, color becomes a part of the process of digestion, ingestion, and oxidization. The power of white light in the form of color must be present at all times or medication is useless. One big disadvantage of color received through medication is the many dangerous side effects attending its use.

Exercise, massage, manipulation, hot mineral baths, and other forms of stimulation also depend upon the chemical action of color to heal and build.

The process of digestion and assimilation of food produces colors from the various elements in the food. If there are deficiencies in our diet or assimilation, there is also a deficiency of color corresponding to the missing element.

There is a constant aura of color around each of us. These colors vary according to the condition of the body. Wherever there is a deficiency of minerals or vitamins, there is also a deficiency in the color aura. These colors are visible to many people. Equipment has recently been devised which enables others to see the aura also.

In using color to promote healing and corrections, white light is projected through films of various colors onto the body to reinforce or intercept the color emanations from the body.

A simple example of this is readily shown. When a person is burned (first, second, or third degree) or has a high fever, there is a surplus of red, which is hydrogen. This is intercepted by projection of blue light which is oxygen. The oxygen and hydrogen combine producing water — perspiration. In the case of the burn, all pain is gone in one hour. A complete healing takes approximately 20 days without scars. This has been demonstrated again and again and can be duplicated by anyone who cares to try it.

Color is the active principal of all vitamins. Below is a partial list of the vitamins thus far known to be required by the body. Other vitamins are present in other colors but research is not complete enough to understand the need for the others. Color therapy replaces the need for additional vitamin pills and formulas. The vitamins interestingly enough, were discovered by the color present in each of them.

Vitamin A is yellow.
All B vitamins are present in the orange and red color.
Vitamin C is lemon.
Vitamin D is violet.
Vitamin E is found in scarlet and magenta.
Vitamin K is indigo.

White light, whether from the sun or an artificial source, contains all the colors as seen in the rainbow (or as seen in an ordinary prism). The true primary colors of white light are red, green, and violet. The secondary colors are yellow (a combination of red and green) and blue, (a combination of green and violet). By combining these five colors in various ways, seven other colors are produced to make twelve in all. (See No. 55).

By the scientific application of color to our bodies, we introduce a natural energy that enables our bodies to eliminate waste and congestion. At the same time, color can repair virtually every form of damage due to injury or sickness.

The scientific application of color is one of the great natural sources of healing. The results that have been achieved have been little short of miraculous.

Truly the Divine science of color healing is a miracle of simplicity. It is neither a fad nor an illusion. It deals with the higher vibratory forces of nature through the source of all power — light.

Since it is the visable rays of the sun that are used for healing purposes, one might suppose that taking sun baths in the nude is the most practical solution. This seems logical, but not quite reasonable. If you believed in medication by drugs, when you became ill would you go to the drug store and buy a combination of all the medicines in the store and then proceed to take them all at once, hoping you might get what you needed? Or would you buy only what you thought you needed?

It is reasonable to take only the corrective you need at the time you need it. In the scientific application of color, we project only what we need at the time we need it. Even if it were feasible to use the rays of the sun directly, one cannot always get the sun when one might need it most. There are often days when we never see the sun (not to mention nights!).

If you should suddenly become ill late in the evening, and help was needed in a hurry, waiting until the next day for the sun to shine is hardly the answer. There are also many days of cold weather — too cold to lie nude for long.

If all the conditions were exactly right, you would get some good from the sun — particularly if you were already tanned to protect yourself from the destructive rays of the sun. Probably the destructive invisible rays would do damage before the healing of the visible rays could take place. But if all the above conditions are just right and little beads of perspiration are present, the white light is broken into its various colors and the body uses only the colors it needs and rejects the rest. Our bodies have the ability to choose only the color they need from the sun, if we are not too depleted.

Getting all the necessary elements from our food is also important. Plants are governed by the same natural law as everything else. They have the ability to pick up just the color and chemicals they need, if all are present in the soil and air where they grow. If a plant becomes sickly from lack of sufficient minerals and water, the sun can do it no good. It takes every natural condition to produce a perfectly healthy plant — or human being. Each vegetable, fruit and flower has an individual color of its own. When we eat any kind of food, we are actually eating color from the sun. The chemicals and minerals are there because of the action of the color in the suns' rays. Of course, the minerals and water have to be in the soil and air or the colors could not make the plant grow.

If we are unable to use the suns' rays directly, we must then resort to other sources of white light and scientific color to assist in the healing process.

In the field of color healing, there is no need to think in terms of several thousand names of diseases. The name is not important; it will heal nothing. Much time and error is involved in determining the name and the type of medication or procedure to follow. Healing with color simplifies the entire procedure. In reality there is but one disease regardless of the name one might call it. The disease is toxemia as we have emphasized before — the accumulation of toxins or poisons in the body. It is divided into two varieties: acute and chronic. All acute diseases are hot diseases; in other words, there is a fever. All chronic diseases are conditions without a fever. All hot (acute) disorders are corrected or balanced by use of the cold colors. All cold (chronic) disorders are corrected or balanced by use of the warm colors. If in doubt as to which color should be used, start with green, the neutral color.

Classification of Colors
— hot or cold —

Hot or Acute Colors	Fulcrum or Neutral Colors	Cold or Chronic Colors
Lemon	Green	Turquoise
Yellow	Magenta	Blue
Orange		Indigo
Red		Violet
Scarlet		Purple

General Directions for Use of Color

Each of the colors has a different effect on the body, yet they are all interrelated. They all work together to relieve, cleanse, build, and heal. There are no dangerous side effects at any time. Only a normal condition can occur regardless of the length of exposure time on the body, face, or eyes. Since the color works through the aura to make the changes, only the amount necessary will ever be accepted; as with a pail of water, only the full amount will be accepted and the rest will overflow. (The bulb used is not a heat lamp; it is the color, not the heat, that does the healing).

If the process of loosening and eliminating the toxins occurs very rapidly, one might feel upset. It is not necessary to stop as no damage is being done. If acute or dizzy conditions develop, turquoise may be used for temporary relief.

Each application of color should be for one hour or more; wait for two hours or more before the next one. Emergency treatments may be taken at any time, day or night, to obtain desired relief. With the possible exception of severe burns, generally speaking, it is needless to continue exposure for several hours at one time. It is always best to stay with about one hour on and two hours or more off. Give the body a chance to make the necessary changes. Continued exposure of hours can possibly stir up more toxins than the eliminative organs can handle at the moment due to the weakened condition or being overworked. It won't cause harm but could cause discomfort. Even with burns long hours are not necessary after the pain leaves.

For most conditions you will be using the warm colors but the cold colors also have many benefits and can be used from time to time just to relax, tone and condition various organs and nerves.

Treatments may be taken at any time before eating, but wait for two hours or more after a meal. If indigestion occurs, however, yellow may be used at the time.

The color has the maximum benefit if applied to the nude body. A cover of a white sheet has lesser effects. Normal light in the room will not interfere with the effect of the color, but do not use in the direct sunlight or other strong lights. It will dissipate the strength of the color. Have the

115

room warm enough to prevent a chill. Since it is the effect of the color and not the heat, the lamp may be four to eight feet from the body. Hang it on the wall or suitable post about five feet above the body. It is best to be in a reclining position or sitting. The swivel on the lamp allows proper exposure on different areas. The base has a small hole in the hook that is suitable for a hook on the wall.

Use of the Twelve Colors

Red:

The longest wave length in the visible spectrum is red.

It is the lowest rate of vibration of the visible spectrum.

It is an outgoing vibration related to aggressiveness and conquest. It is an expression of vitality, of nervousness, and of glandular activity. It is a very exciting color.

A strong, clear red in the aura indicates force, vigor, and energy. It is also the color of warmth, love and tenderness. Treating with this color stimulates the automatic nervous and circulatory systems. A clear dark red is a sensual color, building and stimulating the five senses. It is a very strong selling color. High pressure salesmanship is predominantly red. It is an irritant and excitant.

A dark and cloudy red indicates high temper and nervous turmoil. A light thin red aura indicates a nervous, impulsive, and self-centered person with very little reserve of nervous energy.

Man evolves from the low gross color of red through the entire color spectrum to the highest of colors, violet.

Red projected on the body:

Stimulates and builds the liver.

Builds the red corpuscles in the liver which are stored in the bone marrow for any needed emergency or sudden loss of blood.

Is a pustulant — draws poisons to a head on the surface to be eliminated.

The negative aspect of red is an aggressive warlike attitude and instability with a very strong sex drive.

Orange:

Orange is the color of success. Projected on the body it contributes to the following:

Helps you expand your interests and activities.

Gives life and healing with its increase in oxygen by stimulation of the lungs and thyroid glands.

It depresses the parathyroid glands.

It stimulates the production of milk in the mammary glands. This eliminates the need for animal milks and artificial formulas. Nothing can compare with mother's milk if she is eating the correct foods.

Causes vomiting or stimulates action in the opposite direction in case of indigestion.

Relieves gas in the digestive system; alleviates convulsions and cramps in all parts of the body. It is most effective for hiccups.

Relieves a spastic and sluggish colon and intestines.

Increases all kinds of discharges and eliminations.

Decreases menstrual cramps and increases discharges.

It is a pustulant; drawing boils, carbuncles, and abscesses to a head.

It is a lung builder and respiratory stimulant. It heals all lung disorders.

Most spices come under the orange color and may be used sparingly in the diet. They contain many trace elements that may be lacking in other foods. Black and white pepper must not be used at any time as they contain a form of cumulative poison. Other spices act as a mild laxative and stimulant for the digestive tract.

Yellow:

Yellow is a creative color. It brings the following benefits.

Stimulating, activating, endless energy and building of the motivating actions in the body.

Creates self-confidence and courage.

Depresses the spleen and the parathyroid gland.

Increases the appetite.

Aids in better assimilation for better nutrition.

Stimulates the lymphatic glands.

Acts as a motivating action for all kinds of paralysis such as in strokes or sluggish organs.

Is a nerve stimulant and builder.

Stimulates and strengthens the heart for better circulation.

Stimulates the liver and gall bladder, aiding in better eliminations.

Destroys body worms and drives them out of the body. Worms and insects shy away from the yellow.

Stimulates and builds the pancreas for better control of the sugar balance.

Stimulates and builds the eyes and ears.

Loosens and aids in elimination of calcium and lime deposits that cause arthritis, neuritis and similar conditions.

Yellow is a most inspiring color.

Lemon:

Lemon has more elements than any other color. Projected on the body:

It is a chronic alterative — loosening, relaxing and stimulating the eliminative processes.

Its phosphorus stimulates and builds the brain for clearer and more positive thinking.

Loosens and eliminates mucus throughout the entire body.

Activates and loosens congestion in the colon for better elimination.
Loosens and dissolves calcium and lime deposits.
Activates the thymus gland for better and more rapid growth in
retarded children.
Is a bone builder. It heals broken bones faster and hardens soft
bones.
Is extremely effective for loosening and eliminating the common
cold.
The lemon fruit is the best of all foods to loosen and cleanse. It
contains all the elements in the lemon color plus much more.
Is a soothing color because it relieves tension.

Green:

Green is the master color. It is the fulcrum of the primary colors and
stands out as the key to prepare the body for more effective results from
the other colors:
It stimulates the pituitary, the master gland.
Is a vibrant color of life and growth — the most predominating color
in the life force of our planet.
Is crisp, cool, and fresh-cleansing in nature.
Has the universal appeal to the sense of balance and normality.
Raises the vibrations of the body above the vibrations of disease — a
form of immunity from all disease.
Destroys and heals all infections. Hospitals find less infections when
green is present.
Is the color of clarity — destroying rotting material and building cells
and tissues. This is nitrogen, the substance of protein, the builder of
muscles. Animal proteins are highly toxic and destructive. They have
no place in creative nutrition.
Many elements needed by the body are absorbed from the air through
the lungs. It is recognized that oxygen and hydrogen are taken from the
air, but few realize that nitrogen is also taken from the air and used as a
protein builder. Breathing fresh air and eating of fresh fruits and vegetables eliminates completely any possible need for any of the animal forms
of food.
Smoking prevents the lungs from utilizing the nitrogen from the air.
Heavy smokers have a craving for toxic animal proteins. Plants obtain a
great percentage of their nitrogen from the air also.
Green is the basic color for all disorders of either chronic or acute
conditions. Start all schedules with one or more green exposures. Many
conditions may be cleared up with green alone.
Green dissolves blood clots in any part of the body or head. It takes
less than an hour to accomplish this. There is nothing in medicine that
works so fast. The chemicals used for this purpose have many dangerous
side effects. There are no side effects from the use of green.

The main color used for cancer is green. Cancer feeds on waste and rotting conditions within the body. When these wastes are removed from the body, the cancer cannot feed on healthy tissue, so it breaks up and passes out of the body — absolutely harmlessly. The fear of cancer is greatly exaggerated. The fear of cancer kills more people than the cancer itself.

A clean, healthy body will never produce any form of cancer.

The use of green on open sores, cuts, bruises and damaged flesh is truly wonderful.

Use green for burns in connection with turquoise to build muscle and tissue, and to build new skin without scars. (See turquoise below.)

Turquoise:

Turquoise is an acute alterative for all sudden pains and aches. Use turquoise after the green for all infections.

Use turquoise for skin building when damaged by any degree of burns, scratches, sores and infections. Pain from burns is usually gone within one hour. The complete healing of third degree burns occurs in less than three weeks without a trace of a scar. Use coconut oil on the burned area to keep it soft.

All fevers regardless of the name, are caused by the same thing and respond quickly — usually in one hour. It is a tonic, quickly reviving conditions of fatigue poisons. Work, play and exercise produce these poisons as the cells and tissues are broken down, making one feel tired. Turquoise is very cooling and relaxing — especially for headaches and pressures.

It is for irritations, inflammations, and itching.

It is a mental or brain depressant — especially good for sleeping. Use instead of sleeping pills — a mild sedative with no side effects.

Blue:

The oxygen in blue unites or intercepts the hydrogen in red to increase perspiration as a fever is broken.

It is a vitality builder — the oxygen neutralizes the fatigue poisons for a more relaxed and calming condition.

Blue is the color of the pineal gland, the color of the spirit.

A strong, deep blue in the aura indicates maturity, calmness, and dependability.

A light thin blue in the aura indicates anemia.

Blue is a creative force.

It produces a peaceful effect for sounder sleep.

It relieves itching and irritations.

It relieves all fevers and burns, just slightly stronger than the turquoise — to be used after the turquoise if fever still persists.

Indigo:

Indigo depresses the thyroid and at the same time stimulates the para-thyroid.

It is an analgesic — giving relief especially to pain from extreme swelling. Actually reduces acute swelling as well as relieving the pain.

It is a very strong sedative.

Stops hemorrhages and nose bleeds.

Stops internal bleeding into the tissues and organs.

It is an astringent — tightening, firming and toning the flesh, skin and nerves. (Women particularly enjoy its effect of firming the skin.)

As an antibiotic, it equals or surpasses any of the manufactured products on the market **with no harmful side effects.** The body never becomes allergic or intolerant to its antiseptic action.

Has a narcotic effect — produces a strong, deep sleep. Upon awakening, there are no hangovers or drug-like, effects. Instead, one feels alive, alert, and refreshed.

Depresses the heart; shrinks an enlarged heart.

Violet:

Violet has the shortest wave length of the visible colors.

A motor depressant — depressing all over-active parts of the body except the spleen and the parathyroid.

It is a spiritual color.

Relaxes, calms, and depresses the nerves, as in over excitable people.

It is also an antibiotic, building organisms that destroy harmful organisms.

As a spleenic stimulant it builds the white corpuscles in the spleen. The spleen produces Vitamin D. As the blood passes through the spleen to the heart, a final cleansing takes place to remove any harmful poison or bad cells.

Reduces excitement and extreme irritations.

Depresses the action of the lymphatic glands for lowered nutrition such as in overweight.

Depresses the appetite.

Is a cardiac depressant, relaxing and soothing to the muscles and nerves controlling the heart.

Gives relief from dysentary and diarrhea.

Gives a wonderful deep sleep similar to the Indigo.

Purple:

Purple slows the heart beat and relieves pain and pressure in the heart.
Depresses action in the arteries.
Stimulates the action in veins.
Lowers the blood pressure; relieves pain of headaches and pains from excess pressure.
Depresses overactive kidneys and adrenal glands.
Is a hypnotic — produces relaxed deep sleep with no hangover.
Excellent for calming and putting children to sleep.
Reduces sex desire.
Depresses over-emotional conditions.
Is an excellent color for deep meditation.
Decreases excessive discharges and menstrual pains.
Purple may be interchanged from time to time with turquoise for many types of fevers (such as malaria and rheumatic fevers).

Scarlet:

Scarlet speeds up the heart beat; it strengthens and builds.
Stimulates action in the arteries.
Depresses the veins.
Raises the blood pressure for more alertness.
Stimulates sluggish kidneys and adrenal glands.
Increases and stimulates the emotions.
Scarlet may be interchanged wherever lemon is indicated.
Especially beneficial for congestion and pain in back (lumbago and arthritis).
Increases sluggish menstrual discharges.

Magenta:

Magenta balances the emotions. It is soothing and relaxing both to over-emotional and under-emotional conditions.
Stimulates and builds the heart.
Will produce similar stimulative and depressive effects to those of both scarlet and purple. It works slightly slower.
Will raise or lower the blood pressure automatically to produce a normal condition.
Stimulates or depresses the veins or the arteries for normal function.
Stimulates or depresses the kidneys and adrenal glands.
Balances the sex desires and abilities.
As with green, magenta is used for all disorders and conditions — it makes the other colors more effective.
Builds the aura — strengthens and intensifies.

The Opposing Colors

Red	opposite to	Blue
Orange	opposite to	Indigo
Yellow	opposite to	Violet
Lemon	opposite to	Turquoise
Green	the fulcrum	no opposite
Purple	opposite to	Scarlet
Magenta	the fulcrum	no opposite

Each of the colors work in opposition to each other to balance and create harmony for correct healing. The Magenta and Green have no opposite. They are the fulcrum and effect conditions on both sides of the spectrum.

Color is a Part of Our Daily Life

With color we can create any atmosphere we desire, beginning with the underlying principle of fundamental balance throughout the universe. This creative force produces an awareness of energy beyond the normal range of being. This awareness brings greater abilities and harmony for superior growth.

The colors in our home — the colors we wear, the ones we project, even those in the food we select — determine the path and the progress we make in our goals of achievement.

Our selection of colors determines our acceptance or rejection of others and by others who may or may not harmonize with us.

We absolutely can not live without light and color. The more creatively and sensitively we use it, the more advanced we become physically, mentally, and spiritually. So make the most of the healing qualities of color for a more creative life. It is the essence of the life force all about us.

The application of the colors may be directly on the affected part or parts or on the entire body as needed. If any part of the body has congested or deficient disorders, the rest of the body is also affected. We must always consider the overall picture when correcting any disorder. All colors used singularly or in various combinations can only assist in creating a normal condition. They work automatically to balance all functions. Their use is completely harmless regardless of the length of exposure on any part of the body. Use them in the order they are written.

The figures under "number of applications" indicate the number of treatments to be taken — **each treatment is one hour with two or more hours in between.** Take as many hours each day or night as your time permits. Each schedule may take a week or more.

The number under the area heading indicates the whole area for each application. (No. 56 on page 116).

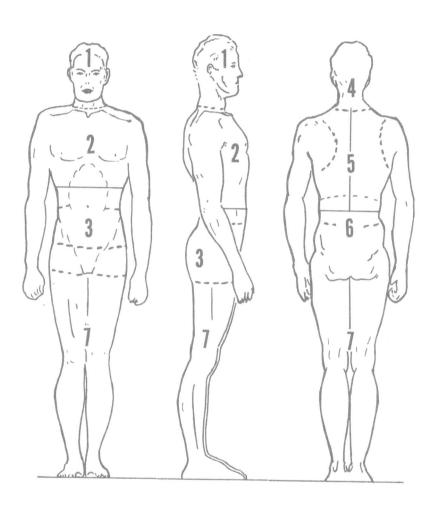

Color Combinations

Primary colors .... red, green, violet
Secondary colors .... yellow and blue
All other colors are combinations of these five

Red		single color
Orange	combine	red and yellow
Yellow		single color
Lemon	combine	yellow and green
Green		single color
Turquoise	combine	blue and green
Blue		single color
Indigo	combine	blue and violet
Violet		single color
Scarlet	combine	red and blue
Purple	combine	· violet and yellow
Magenta	combine	red and violet

Schedules

To help you make the transition from the name of disease to the understanding of the condition being either hot or cold, I have prepared the following schedules. The cold condition is a congestion. The hot condition is a release of the congestion and its eliminative effects.

Schedules

1. For all degrees of burns. Use the same schedule for open or decaying sores on body or limbs.

Number of applications	Color	Area
2	Turquoise	Affected part
2	Green	Affected part
2	Green	1-2-3
1	Magenta	4

Continue alternating with the Green and Turquoise until completely healed. If other conditions need correcting, use the other needed colors' occasionally.

2. Boils, Abscesses, Carbuncles, Eczema and all types of weeping or dry sores anywhere on the body.

Number of applications	Color	Area
3	Green	1-2-3
2	Magenta	2
2	Magenta	5
2	Lemon	1-2-3 or locally
2	Orange	1-2-3 or locally

Conclude with two or more applications of yellow as needed to complete the elimination of all discharges. After all discharges have stopped, use Turquoise and Indigo alternately until healing is complete.

3. Cancer, Leukemia, and Tumors.

Number of applications	Color	Area
5	Green	1-2-3
3	Magenta	2
3	Magenta	6
3	Lemon	1-2-3
3	Yellow	1-2-3
5	Green	1-2-3
3	Magenta	1-2-3
3	Magenta	6

Repeat as needed.

Since cancer, Leukemia, and tumors are caused by masses of toxic waste and deficiencies, the Lemonade Diet may be used several times to great advantage. Eat plenty of green foods.

Schedules (Cont.)

4. Varicose Veins, Hemorrhoids, Glaucoma, Phlebitis, and similar conditions.

Number of applications	Color	Area
3	Green	1-2-3
3	Green	Locally
2	Magenta	2
2	Magenta	6
3	Purple	Locally
3	Indigo	Locally

Repeat as needed.

5. Colds, Influenza, Swine flu, Measles, Whooping Cough, Scarlet Fever, and all Pneumonia and Bronchial disorders. All acute disorders come under this schedule.

Number of applications	Color	Area
3	Green	1-2-3

If fever is present, alternate first with Turquoise and then with Blue. If no fever, or when broken, use:

Number of applications	Color	Area
3	Lemon	1-2-3
3	Yellow	1-2-3
3	Magenta	2
2	Magenta	6
2	Orange	1-2-3
2	Red	1-2-3

Repeat if necessary.

6. Eyes, Ears and Nose.

Number of applications	Color	Area
2	Magenta	2
2	Magenta	6
1	Green	1
2	Lemon	1
4	Yellow	1
8	Orange	1
16	Red	1

Repeat if necessary.

Schedules (Cont.)

7. Multiple Sclerosis, Arthritis, Rheumatism, Bursitis, Neuritis, and other similar conditions.

Number of applications	Color	Area
4	Green	1-2-3
2	Magenta	2
2	Magenta	6
4	Lemon	On affected part
5	Yellow	On affected part
2	Magenta	2
2	Magenta	6
2	Orange	1-2-3

If pain increases or fever develops, use Turquoise or Indigo for temporary relief.

8. Constipation, Diabetes, all forms of Paralysis.

Number of applications	Color	Area
3	Green	1-2-3
3	Lemon	2-3
3	Magenta	2
2	Magenta	6
3	Yellow	2-3

Repeat as needed.

9. All forms of Anemia and Heart trouble.

Number of applications	Color	Area
3	Green	1-2-3
3	Lemon	2-3
3	Yellow	2-3
2	Magenta	2
2	Magenta	6
5	Red	3
1	Violet	3
5	Red	3

Repeat as needed.

Schedules (Cont.)

10. Asthma, Hay Fever, Sinus, and all similar conditions.

TO BREAK ANY FEVER: Turquois for one hour; — if fever still continues, use Blue followed by Indigo.

Number of applications	Color	Area
3	Green	1-2
3	Lemon	3
3	Magenta	2
3	Magenta	6
3	Orange	1-2
1	Indigo	1
3	Green	1-2
2	Magenta	1-2
2	Magenta	6
2	Lemon	1-2
2	Yellow	3

Repeat as needed.

11. Tuberculosis, Emphysema, and Chronic Lung conditions such as Cystic Fibrosis.

Number of applications	Color	Area
3	Green	1-2-3
2	Lemon	3
2	Magenta	2
2	Magenta	6
6	Lemon	1-2
6	Orange	1-2
3	Yellow	3
6	Orange	1-2

Repeat as needed.

12. Muscular Dystrophy ("Dystrophy" means imperfect or faulty nutrition according to Webster's dictionary).

Number of applications	Color	Area
6	Green	1-2-3
3	Magenta	2
3	Lemon	1-2-3
3	Yellow	1-2-3
3	Orange	1-2-3
5	Red	1-2-3

Repeat as needed.

128

SPECIAL NOTE: Over the last decade many millions of dollars have been collected (and presumably spent) for research. So far the answer is always: "We still don't know — give us more money to fight this crippling disease." Yet there it is right in the dictionary — Faulty Diet. All that is needed is correct diet (read the Master Cleanser) as we have demonstrated again and again in our work.

Is it necessary for the American public to be systematically "conned" by the big rip-off of yearly donations for research? The cause and correction is already here.

The above schedules may be changed or varied to suit each case. All chronic disorders are brought to an acute state for elimination from the body. This is Nature's way to free us from our disease-producing toxins. Germs and Viruses are the Creator's gift to assist in cleaning the body of pollution.

The simplest and most effective method of applying the colors is with a small lamp built in this fashion: Start with a swivel base with a three-inch standard socket to hold a 150 watt reflector spot bulb (as used for indoor lighting). Prepare an outer hood to cover the bulb enough to focus the light ahead. The hood must have enough open space in the back for good ventilation. This prevents the bulb and colors from burning out too quickly. This may be mounted on the wall by hook or on a movable standard about 7 feet tall.

The most effective and balanced type of color is produced by projecting through plastic sheets. They must be so balanced that when the three primary colors of Red, Green and Violet are projected from separate lamps on a white screen, white light is produced. Balanced yellow with blue completes the five colors that are used to make the remaining colors. (A framework to hold the colored plastic sheets needs to be attached to the lamp hood.)

Read the general directions over again and follow instructions carefully.

For information about obtaining a color lamp contact: VITA-GEM ENTERPRISES, VICTORIA, B.C., CANADA. **(250) 388-4102**

Elements According to Color Classification

Red:
Cadmium
Hydrogen
Krypton
Neon

Orange:
Aluminum
Antimony
Arsenic
Boron
Calcium
Copper
Helium
Selenium
Silicon
Xenon

Yellow:
Beryllium
Carbon
Iridium
Magnesium
Molybdenum
Osmium
Palladium
Platinum
Rhodium
Ruthenium
Sodium
Tin
Tungsten

Lemon:
Cerium
Germanium
Gold
Iodine
Iron
Lanthanum
Neodymium
Phosphorus
Praseodymium
Samarium
Scandium
Silver
Sulphur
Thorium
Titanium
Uranium
Vanadium
Yttrium
Zirconium

Green:
Barium
Chlorine
Nitrogen
Radium
Tellurium
Thallium

Turquoise:
Chromium
Fluorine
Mercury
Nickel
Niobium
Tantalum
Zinc

Blue:
Caesium
Indium
Oxygen

Indigo:
Bismuth
Lead
Polonium
Thorium

Violet:
Actinium
Cobalt
Gallium
Radon

Purple:
Bromine
Europium
Gadolinium
Terbium

Magenta:
Lithium
Potassium
Ribidium
Strontium

Scarlet:
Argon
Dysprosium
Erbium
Holmium
Lutetium
Manganese
Thulium
Ytterbium

Biochemistry

Essential Salts

Calcium	Effects	Principal Containing Foods	
Bone and Heart	Builds and maintains bone	Cress 35	Whey 13*
Mineral Daily	structures; gives	Dill 31	Milk 12*
Need,	vitality, endurance;	Cabbage 21	Onion 10
648-972 mg.	anti-acid	Chard 21	Carrots 7
		Radish 15	Grapes 2

Sodium			
Ligaments,	Aids digestion; counter-	Celery 65	Lettuce 13
Heart, Blood,	acts acidity; purifies	Spinach 62	Cucumber . 10
Secretions,	blood, halts fermenta-	Chard 62	Beets 9
3.89-5.83 gm.	tion; preserves youth-	Tomato 32	Bananas 6
	fulness.	Carrots 14	Prunes 3

Phosphorus			
Brain and Bone	Nourishes brain and	Kale 35	Cucumber . 10
mineral.	nerves; builds power of	Bran 27	Spinach 18
2.92-3.89 gm.	thought; stimulates growth	Radish 23	Lettuce 16
	of hair and bones	Pumpkin ... 23	Milk 15*

Sulphur			
Brain and Tissue	Purifier: tones system;	Kale 86	Turnip 12
Salt.	Intensifies feeling and	Cress 53	Parsnip 8
1.94-3.24 gm.	emotion; gives versa-	Dill 20	Chard 6
	tility	Cabbage 17	Lettuce 6
		Beans 12	Carrots 4
		Spinach 12	H'radish 35

Chlorine			
For the Heart	With Potassium, Calcium	Cheese 26*	Beets 9
and Secretions.	and Sodium, it controls	Dill Tea 14	Milk 8*
Blood Cleanser	the heart beat. Expels	Lettuce 13	Cress 7
	body wastes; cleanser.	Whey 11*	Avocado 6
		Cabbage 10	Molasses ... 6

Magnesium			
Nerve Mineral	Relaxes nerves; cools	Tomato 13	Cucumber . 4
324-518 mg.	and relieves brain lag;	Spinach 11	Figs 3
	laxative, refreshes;	Lettuce 11	Carrots 3
	motor stimulant.	Bran 9	Walnuts 2
		Celery 6	Oranges 2
		Beans 6	Grapefruit . 1

*The foods marked thus * are given here merely as a comparison and not for good nutrition.*

Biochemistry

Essential Salts

Silicon
Nails, Skin,
Hair, Teeth.
6.48 mg.

Effects
Makes tissues supple;
Gives grace, litheness,
keen hearing, sparkling
eyes, hard teeth,
glossy hair.

Principal Containing Foods

Lettuce	14	Beets	7
Asparagus .	9	Chard	5
Dandelion .	0	Celery	4
Onions	8	Cherries	3
Spinach	8	Figs	2
Cucumber .	8		

Iron
Corpuscles of
Blood.
12.96 mg.

Absorbes oxygen and
feeds tissues; gives
vitality; rosy cheeks,
vigor; brings blood
count up.

Sorrel	9	Onions	1
Lettuce	9	Artichoke ..	1
Leeks	7	Watermelon	1
Spinach	6	Cucumber .	1
Radish	3	Tomato	1
Str'berry	3		

Manganese
Cell, Memory,
Strength.
A trace.

Resistance to disease,
coordinates thought
and action, raises
blood pressure;
heart stimulant.

Peppermint leaves, Nasturtium
leaves, Almonds, Walnuts,
Parsley, Wintergreen, Bran.

Flourine
Tooth Enamel,
Bone Preserver.
Trace.

Acute alterative, skin
builder; strengthens
tendons, knits bones,
improves eyes.

Cabbage, Cauliflower, Goat's*
Milk, Spinach, Tomatoes,
Cress, Juniper Berries.

Iodine
Gland, Brain,
Beauty. Trace.

Prevents goiter,
loosens congestion,
ejects poisons.

Sea lettuce, carrots, pineapple, garlic, potato skins,
avocado.

(Figures represent number of mineral parts contained in 1000 parts of food.)
(1 gm. − 1 gram = 1000 mg., = 1000 milligrams)

*The foods marked thus * are given here merely as a comparison and not for good nutrition.*

Biochemistry

High Sodium (Na) Foods	Na	K
Celery	65	49
Spinach	63	29
Swiss Chard	62	44
Romaine	62	46
Chinese Lettuce	32	16
Beets, Red	21	8
Collards	20	14
Strawberries	19	13
Squash	17	13
Pumpkin	16	12
Pomegranate	16	8
Potato, Sweet	15	13
Bread, Rye*	11	5
Figs, Dry	10	10
Lemons	15	90

High Potassium (K) Foods	K	Na
Kale	81	5
Lettuce	67	13
Turnips	59	7
Dandelion	50	13
Cabbage	45	11
Watercress	44	17
Parsley	41	2
Cucumbers	41	10
Cauliflower	40	5
Beets, White	38	9
Parsnip	33	1
Brussel Sprouts	31	1
Potato, Irish	26	1
Carrots	25	14
Celery Root	22	1
Whey	21	10*
Prunes	18	3
Bananas	16	6
Papaya	9	9
Lemons	90	15

Average Foods

	Na	K
Legumes*	8	159
Nuts*	3	60
Vegetables	165	353
Fruits	16	117

	K	Na
Bread, Grains	8	59
Sugar, White	0	0
Milk & Dairy Products*	56	116

A diet high in sodium foods helps to prevent old age, stones in the body, tumor growths, rheumatism and all hardening processes.

An excess of alkaline sodium over the acid in the blood is known as the "alkaline reserve" and this margin is of utmost importance to vital health.

Heart, Kidney and arterial disorders generally indicate a potassium deficiency.

*These foods are acid-forming, the same as are all forms of meat, fish and eggs; they should be avoided. Most disorders are the result of an over-acid condition.

Biochemistry

Alkaline Foods		Acid Forming	Acid Foods
Figs	Parsley	All Grain Products	All Berries
Bananas	Green Peppers	White Sugar	Pomegranates
Prunes	Lettuce	All Meats	Grapefruit
Raisins	Cabbage	Animal Fats	Persimmon
Dates	Tomatoes	Butter	Pineapple
Avocado	Mustard Greens	Cream	Currants
Grapes	Cucumbers	Eggs	Cherries
Pears	String Beans	Cheese	Oranges
All Potatoes	Green Peas	Sea Foods	Cumquats
Molasses	Sweet Pea	Most Nuts	Peaches
Coconut	Sweet Corn	Dry Beans	Apricots
All Melon	Bean Sprouts	Dry Peas	Quince
Celery	Radishes	Most Oils	Lemons
Spinach	Carrots	Lentils	Apples
Chard	Watercress		Melons
Chinese Lettuce	Pumpkin		Other fruits
Beets	Squash		
Okra			

All acid foods are alkaline in reaction when digested, except in some cases where the body is extremely over acid and the acid foods cannot properly digest; then they often create more acid. When this condition exists, eat alkaline foods until an excess of alkaline balance is obtained, then the acid foods again may be eaten and properly digested.

All acid fruits, berries, and melons are alkaline reacting when normal digestion is present. If the diet consists of fruits, vegetables, berries, seeds and nuts in limited amounts, there is little possibility of indigestion.

Remember — even the best of foods can cause indigestion and imbalances if over-eating is a problem.

Element	(Symbol)	Optimal Daily Intake		Functions &/or Miscellaneous Information
Sodium	(Na)	1150-5800	mg.	Helps regulate body fluid levels.
Potassium	(K)	1900-5870	mg.	Essential for muscle and nerve function.
Calcium	(Ca)	1000-2000	mg.	Most abundant mineral-bones & teeth, nerve & muscle function.
Phosphorus	(P)	1500-3000	mg.	Essential for all chemical reactions, component all tissue.
Magnesium	(Mg)	485-1220	mg.	Essential for activating many enzymes for metabolizing carbohydrates & proteins, balances Ca, hardens teeth & bones.
Chlorine	(Cl)	1770-8860	mg.	
Iron	(Fe)	15-25	mg.	Essential component of hemoglobin (in red blood cells) and other enzymes involved in oxygen transport and use.

Element	(Symbol)	Optimal Daily Intake		Functions &/or Miscellaneous Information
Zinc	(Zn)	15-30	mg.	Essential component of many enzymes in body tissues — especially the sex organs, also important in healing wounds, counteracts cadmium poisoning.
Silicon	(Si)	about 6.5	mg.	Probably essential but function unknown.
Manganese	(Mn)	2-9	mg.	Essential for oxygen transport and the metabolism of fats, carbohydrates, and proteins, promotes sex hormone production.
Copper	(Cu)	1.5-5.0	mg.	Essential component of enzymes that transport oxygen, helps iron absorption, activates other enzymes too.
Fluorine	(F)	1.4-1.8	mg.	Essential component of teeth and bone, small amounts protect against dental decay.
Vanadium	(V)	about 2	mg.	Reduces cholesterol, levels in body, probably essential for fat metabolism.
Iodine	(I)	114-357	μg.	Essential component of thyroid hormones, and seems to help fight infections such as TB.
Chromium	(Cr)	30-100	μg.	Essential for sugar and fat metabolism, probably essential for proper insulin function.
Molybdenum	(M0)	trace		Essential activator of several enzymes.
Cobalt	(C0)	5-8	μg.	Essential component of vitamin B-12 and red blood cells.
Selenium	(Se)	trace		Small amounts essential to help body use vitamin E and metabolise sulfur-containing proteins.
Sulfur	(S)	?		Essential component of all foods, all body tissues.
Boron	(B)	⎫		
Lithium	(Li)	⎬ ?		Probably essential but function unknown.
Strontium	(Sr)	⎪		
Tin	(Sn)	⎭		

Note: 1 gram = 1000 mg. = 1,000,000 μg.; (mg. = **milligram**, μg. = **microgram**)

Element	Some sources of the element
Co	Best sources: sea vegetation. Traces found in all vegetables and fruits.
Cr	Grain cereals, corn. Traces present in fruits and vegetables.
Cu	Whole grains, almonds, green leafy vegetables, dry legumes, sea vegetation.
Mo	Legumes, cereal grains, some dark-green leafy vegetables — depends on soil content.
Se	Bran & germ of cereal grains, some vegetables — broccoli, onions, tomatoes.
V	Sea vegetations are best sources, some in vegetables.
Zn	Whole grains, wheat bran and germ, high protein foods.

Make Your Living More Complete with Color

For those who like color for spot lighting or to accentuate many beautiful appointments in the home, one or more of the color projectors can bring glamour and beautiful tones into your life. The warm colors have stimulating qualities, while the cold colors are cooling and refreshing.

Colors for the walls and ceiling of the home will vary with the use of each room. The warm colors, such as red, orange, yellow, lemon and scarlet, may be used most successfully in the kitchen, dining room, and many types of work quarters. They are stimulating and exciting colors. They are most successful in play rooms because they are creative in principle. The colors express joy and warmth of feeling.

The cool colors, such as turquoise, blue, indigo, violet, and purple, are relaxing, soothing and conducive to sleep. Use these colors in the bedroom, sitting room and den.

White is a combination of all twelve colors and may be used to great advantage in making a room lighter and cleaner looking. However, other colors should be used with white to create variety.

Black is the absence of all color and should never be used for any purpose. Black produces disease, old age and death and should never be worn. Both men and women should shun all black clothing as if it were a plague. The true seeker of health will use only the many shades of the visible colors in his or her attire. The warmer shades are always best because most people express the various shades of the cool colors in their auras and must be balanced with the warm colors.

Green and Magenta may be used whenever or wherever desired as they are neither hot or cold, but are the Fulcrum or balance between the two. They both have the same rate of vibration, so the colors are the same in effect. The apparent difference is that green is a physical color while the Magenta is an emotional or spiritual color. They appear to be different because the waves move in opposite directions as they travel through space. The green moves in a clockwise direction, while the magenta moves counter-clockwise. Some plants have leaves which are green on one side and magenta on the other. There is also a material which appears green one moment and magenta the next as it changes its position.

Add color to your life for Living Creatively!

CHAPTER VI:

Summary and Conclusion

Each separate part of this three-fold system can and does work independently, producing remarkable results entirely by itself. When all three of these systems work together and in harmony with our physical, mental, and spiritual bodies, **absolutely nothing can compare with the ensuing speed and perfection in healing!**

THE MASTER CLEANSER or LEMONADE DIET, coupled with continuing proper nutrition, cleanses and builds for superior health. A sound diet free from animal toxins consists of fruits, vegetables, berries, seeds, nuts, sprouted seeds, and grains. With such a regime freedom from all diseases becomes a reality. One must also understand that these natural foods reach their highest peak of perfection when used in limited amounts. It is never necessary to stuff oneself to supply all of the needed nutrients. Use as much variety of foods as possible. Eat something different every day, but closely follow the mono diet; i.e., when eating fruit, limit yourself to fruit. The same principle works better also for vegetables. An occasional mixture of raw vegetables in a salad with an avocado, nuts, or raisins is not a serious breach of the principle, however.

Raw foods are always superior to cooked. Hippocrates said, "Let your food be your medicine and your medicine be your food." Modern medicine has strayed far from his insight. The use of color therapy renews and revives the ability of the body to properly use the chemical action of food within our body. It stimulates and enhances all body functions, thus coordinating perfectly with the dietary program.

THE REFLEX SYSTEM works in a manner superior to any of the manipulative systems — without exception. Corrections are constantly made that the other systems are unable to duplicate or improve upon.

COLOR THERAPY is truly a miracle of healing with its utilization of natural chemistry. It accelerates and completes the other two approaches.

A Modern Miracle

I would like to describe a perfect example of this trinity in action by citing a recent case. D. Bugbee, approximately 26 years old, was thrown many feet from a moving car in an accident. His head hit a rock and a severe concussion followed. The attending doctor decided there were blood clots. Whereupon holes were drilled in the skull and drainage occurred. Complete paralysis over the entire left side resulted. Little hope remained for recovery, or even for life.

The doctor wanted to cut the skull open and operate on the brain. D. B. probably would not survive the operation — but he wouldn't live anyway, so why not operate?

His mother refused to allow the operation and he was immediately removed from the hospital — a seemingly hopeless cripple.

Night and day use of color began. Daily application of Vita-Flex began. The lemonade diet began and continued for twenty days.

After only 12 days D. B. was able to walk briskly into the doctor's office, completely healed with no side effects. The cost; only $60.00. All of his friends who saw him after the accident and then after the 12 days of treatment were completely astounded. Another miracle of the finest in healing!

The doctor was almost speechless with this modern miracle before his eyes. His best explanation was simply "You are young and had a strong desire to live".

The hospital and doctor's records are there and the facts can be verified. Many friends are available for verification.

This is not a rare case. Thousands have received similar results and many thousands more will continue to have this service available to them through its proponents around the world.

139

The True Story of Dr. J.

At the end of a healing lecture one night I talked with a Dr. J. I asked him if he intended to take my class. His response was "No, but I'll make a deal with you. I am a surgeon, but for some time now I have had to discontinue operating." His hands were all cracked, swollen, and painful. Wearing gloves to operate was no longer possible. "If you will heal my hands I will come to take your class". He had tried everything in the medical field and nothing had worked.

The simplicity of the lemonade diet, plus applications of vinegar on the hands, resulted in a normal condition returning in three weeks. True to his word, he came with his nurse and learned the work.

No More Pills

Mr. S. C. had many serious troubles: Limited ability to move about because of a angina condition; constant pain from a long-standing stomach ulcer; high blood pressure; back pains — and much more in addition to being overweight.

His doctor told him he would have to take a multiplicity of pills the rest of his life.

With our system no tests were made, no diagnosis, no examinations, and few questions. He immediately started the lemonade diet and threw away all daily pills of a large variety. In thirty days there was a loss of thirty pounds with no further aches, pains, or former troubles — and no side effects.

His wife also had many long-standing health problems. These were all corrected with the same method during the same period.

Mr. S. C. had many close friends with a variety of troubles who were introduced to our methods, and all conditions were corrected in a few days. They all followed the lemonade diet and reflex massage system.

Jill's "Hopeless" Condition

Jill came to me while I owned the health club. She walked with much difficulty using two canes and her husband's arm. She appeared very old and decrepit, although she was actually a young woman. Her ailment: Multiple Sclerosis for many years. Prior to coming to me, she had taken weekly treatments for two years from a local chiropractor. The condition had become worse instead of improving. She was apparently a hopeless case.

Six months later with the help of the lemonade diet, Vita-Flex, and color, normal health returned. She became young, vibrant, and very active with no limitations.

Another Modern Miracle

Mr. K. brought his blind wife in one day — her condition also dreaded "M.S.". She had been blind for several years.

The very first reflex massage with color brought about a miracle. As the massage progressed I told her she was going to be able to see normally. Her husband said, "We don't expect that." I replied, "We will see". In minutes she exclaimed, "I can see your eyes — they are blue. Oh! I can see everything." She returned a number of times for further treatments. **All conditions became normal within two months.**

Joe's Exciting Story

Joe, an American Indian, came in one day to see if he could get help. He had been a diabetic for thirty years, was almost totally blind — a very serious terminal case. He was expected to die any day. He hadn't been able to work for ten years.

Joe was using 60 units of insulin daily. The morning I met him he had not taken the dosage yet. He started with the lemonade, color therapy, and reflex massage immediately. No further insulin was needed from the beginning. At no time during the treatments was there any show of sugar in the urine or surplus in the blood. Gradually his eyes returned to normal and in three months he was living a normal life with a steady, well-paying job. His limitations no longer existed. There were no dangerous side effects at any time.

The Real Enemy

Medicine uses germs and viruses as the enemy that must be destroyed-killed-in order for one to get well while ignoring the true facts that the real enemy is toxins-pollution-within the body and must be removed before the victim can find normal health. Killing those harmless critters with poison drugs can only add more toxins, more misery and more diseases which can only require endless treatments which resolves nothing that produces normal health or freedom from diseases.

Competition is the spark of quality and improvement in all businesses and the arts – brings out the best in the millions of participants, but somewhere along the way a good idea got lost in a fanatical move for power and wealth to dictate and control the form of treatment – with no hope for a cure, by the Medical autocracy. Sadness now rules the world of the sick as hope fades endlessly for more than treatments or a variety of needless loss of parts as the scalpel separates many needed God-given parts from a sickly body.

There are millions – out there today – bound by drugs and medical practices – practicing on them with false methods that keep them in pain and misery with endless treatments until they are released from their wasted bodies – and the sad part of it is that the law allows it and promotes it.

When one becomes sick the quality of service should be the very best as designed according to the original needs of the body as designed by our Creator.

Medicine is sadly lacking in this quality since the needs of the body do not include drugs, poison shots, antibodies of foreign design, destructive radiation, or unnatural chemicals that can only produce dangerous side effects that often bring more unwanted changes. If Medicine knew what they were doing there would be no further need for wasteful tests and endless research.

Medicine is always coming up with something new but that something new is still the same old repeat of newer and stronger drugs with more threatening diseases with no correct answers.

There is a killer in our land and it is not cancer, Aids or a variety of other diseases but the dispensers of drugs – legal or illegal – and those with cutting ways.

Diseases do not require killing. They require only the removal of the cause.

If parts or areas are mal-functioning because of congestions or growths, there is logical reason. When finding that reason and removing it naturally with a cleansing diet the surgery is no longer needed or wanted. Only the ignorant resort to surgery for faulty functioning.

Drugs, of any nature, releases the natural body controls of protection from negative effects, penetrating the aura to allow the lower entities of former addicts to enter into and receive similar effects as in their former life on the earth plane.

Many of our criminal elements are invaded by these entities bringing situations beyond the control of the host with many devastating effects on the rest of society. There are no differences between the illegal drugs and the legal drugs as prescribed by Medical standards, in their side effects, and yet the law permits the use of one and denies the other which requires a great deal of tolerance to accept, in the minds of the logical world.

Does a Medical doctors consider themselves so close to the Divine that they can take an unsafe drug and make it safe for healing purposes? An unsafe drug does not change its normal action just because anyone prescribes it or uses it. Surely, Medicine resembles nothing close to the Divine since it is riddled with drugs and dangerous ways.

One may have all the degrees, titles and licenses, in the world, but if one does not have the simple knowledge of cause and effect with correction of all diseases, one has nothing, at all, but sick people who never get well or free from their afflictions.

There is this legacy, handed down by the Medical profession, year after year: They want to justify their right of being by treating the sick with degrading drugs, chemicals, injections, of false needs, and surgeries that deprive the sick of their God given parts.

If this is really all that some people want that is fine for them but there is something so much better for the enlightened because it is completely drug free and fear free of all diseases that still remain a mystery to the medical heresy.

The freedom to choose any form of correction is the moral right of all people with no interference by any government agency regardless of what reason. As a child I saw the Osteopath, the Chiropractor do their thing with many Limitations as well as with Medicine and their many dangerous limitations and I wondered why. Can this be all there is to healing that brings only temporary relief and endless suffering until death brings on the desired release? I saw the fallacies and errors of pills and potions in dosing-doping-a body full of drugs-poisons and shots causing a variety of new and old diseases. If Medicine really knew what they were doing there would be no further need for research into the unknown and endless tests.

The public has absolutely no protection against the many detrimental damages that the medical Doctors and the greedy surgeons do to them with their prescription drugs and needless surgery. There are many records – on file – of thousands of needless deaths from those drugs – no different than the illegal drugs – , faulty diagnosis, causing the victims to commit suicide and allow surgery that destroys and kills. These tragedies occur because there is no law that protects the victims from dangerous practices.

Just because a Doctor has a medical degree and a license to practice it does not qualify him to treat because – as he says – he is still practicing as he knows so little of the natural needs of the body. With this situation, in mind, the public must realize that we have a life and death situation in – so called, health actions running wild with no controls or no health principals that are naturally required to produce and retain normal healthy living that should pass the quality standards of the divine direction. This is quite obvious or there would not be so many terminally ill people dying from ignorance of the true needs of the body in this age of great advances in technology in other sciences for greater enlightenment of more abundant living instead of millions of agonizing deaths yearly. It is really tragic that medical-drug-doctors and surgery are allowed and promoted-by-law-to continue their evil and ignorant ways at such a high cost of finances, life and death.

Why should one go to a medical doctor for treatments for life while there is corrections available, for your conditions for a short period of time? Honestly now – wouldn't you – all of you rather have fast and simple correction to endless and questionable drug treatments that cost so much in money and misery?

The use of drugs – for any disease – does not – never does – produce the desired results – if your desire is for correction instead of relief because of the many dangerous side effects because none of the drugs were never a part of the original natural makeup of the body.

Many people go to Mexico or other countries for a variety of drugs described as curing a variety of diseases. But drugs never cure anything whether prescribed here or there and so the search goes on for the lack of the the realities. The more that medicine changes the more it remains the same dangerous drugs, expensive needless surgery and lack of credible practices.

Why is a medical doctor permitted to dispense dangerous drugs while others are not?

Medical drugs – as dangerous as other drugs – have the same ability to addict and destroy the lives of those that use them for a variety of diseases – through ignorance – of those trusted falsely to heal those mysterious ills.

Within the realms of unresolved healing the remnants of the ages of questionable magic drugs and potions have been expanded to encompass a never ending supply of needless, useless and more dangerous elixers lacking in the qualities most needed for natural nutritional needs thus retaining the original symptoms and complaints plus volumes of more dangerous undesirables.

It is realistically logically that the most important thing, in the mind of the sick, is that they be allowed to use the very best of healing regardless of from where it comes. There are several million people, out there, lacking the quality of healing that is required to bring fast and accurate healing because the Medical Doctors only treat them with a large variety of drugs that do not heal but become addictive instead. These drugs are foreign to the needs of the body with many needless side effects that only delay the due process of natural healing. Why should the people be shackled-enslaved-by such a system of questionable nature, lacking the validity of natural healing?

Why should a Medical Doctor be given immunity to prosecution while promoting drugs while other dispensers of natural methods are given the full benefits of legal punishment?

If others should discover better more logical ways – more natural ways – the right ways – to completely heal the body quickly with absolutely no side effects, is there any logical reason why this system, should not be accepted instead of being condemned and squashed because it is contrary to accepted practices?

The days of miracles are not over, you can be healed but not by drugs or surgery but by the natural power within working knowingly with the Universal Mind. It is practically impossible to believe that the Medical system should be protected by law while there are superior systems available to the sick that are being condemned by law.. The proof of this statement can very easily be found if the authorities care enough to investigate the truth.

The lack of credibility in Medical practices lacks the quality of healing that is desirable and necessary for those that require the best in natural healing. Their entire procedures are completely ridiculous as their approach to corrections or a "cure" is based on false actions that only complicate the illnesses. Medicine uses germs and viruses as the enemy that must be destroyed-killed-in order for anyone to get well while ignoring the true facts that the real enemies are toxins-pollutions-within the body and must be removed before the drugs can only add more toxins, more suffering and more diseases requiring endless treatments which resolves nothing that produces any form of corrections or free-dom from diseases because the cause has not been eliminated. Germs and viruses are not the causes of our diseases – they are the result. Diseases do not require killing – they require the preservation of life by cleansing out the pollutions and rebuilding the deficiencies with live foods instead of drugs.

Special protection so often breeds contempt for life as it deteriorates from its original purpose of quality healing.

The ancients, living close to nature and to the earth considered nature divine as opposed to tampering with the unknown and unproven manipulating with the artificial which have proven the least likely to qualify as an effective form of healing quality.

People fear that which they do not understand or they accept by ignoring the facts with complete faith hoping no harm can come from its being. This applies to all things – old or new – where ignorance dwells in the minds of the uninformed.

Ignorance is the pathway to sickness and death in the healing field and ignorance abounds in the medical field of practices as the millions of sickly struggle blindly through the endless confusion of faith in drugs that perform as only drugs can perform – in a manner that degrades and disqualifies them from being realistic in restoring normal health. Igno-rance is the essence in standard medical procedures lacking the ability to sustain life to its highest level. The entities involved and the side effects knows no difference between the legal and illegal drugs. They are all accepted as equally as undesirable and unneeded for normal health.

Medicine uses fear in many ways to take and keep control of the sick. Fear comes from ignorance by using false causes of diseases with unsolved corrections since those mysterious unseen-normal sight-critters are falsely charged, poisoned-drugged-or interferred with vaccine or blasted with unnatural shots with dangerous side effects which have created new and more devastating diseases while often retaining the original complaints. Thus the patient and their intended benefactors-the critters-are forced to suffer unnecessary agonies through ignorance. Can medicine really be that ignorant or are they just playing stupid to gain and keep control of the masses through sickness?

As we are entering the new age of enlightenment it is only fitting and proper that we begin to accept only the best of all possible knowledge in healing as well as the finest in spiritual experiences and work knowingly with these principles for our greatest benefits.

It is a proven fact that drugs, of any nature, are foreign to the natural needs or original chemistry of the healthy body.

Drugs are the favorite Medical stock in trade. Drugs always respond as drugs are designed to respond, as addictive and degenerative contrary to the normal and original needs of the physical and mental requirements of a healthy life. Learn to know the difference between drugs and nourishing foods. Learn to say no to drugs in your search for freedom in quality living.

Drugs are a large variety of lies . . . in their wait for their victims.

Drugs – are the favorite medical stock in trade. Drugs always respond as drugs are designed to respond, as addictive and degenerative contrary to the normal and original needs of the physical and mental requirements of a healthy life. Learn to know the difference between drugs and nourishing foods. Learn to say no to drugs in your search for freedom in quality living. Drugs are a large variety of lies . . . in wait for their victims.

A STRIKING EXAMPLE OF DRUG SIDE EFFECTS AS PRESCRIBED BY MEDICAL PRACTICES

A drug that was prescribed by medical doctors for pregnant women to help them sleep and relax or perhaps just to prescribe, is Thalidomide. Over the years, many mal-formed children were born without arms or legs to suffer a lifetime of many handicaps while their parents and friends suffered with them. No legal action was taken against the offenders. WHY?

Mercy killing does occur to some extent but death from faulty diagnoses and faulty prescriptions - drugs - occur far too often but no legal action is taken against such practices. This is standard medical procedures.

A Final Word

This three-fold system accepts no limitations as **to the ability of the human body to heal itself.** I feel so strongly about this work that I am compelled to add a personal touch to bring it all together.

Over the years, since this work came to me, a steady flow of "hopeless" cases have come to find help, relief, and correction. Usually they found much more than they expected and went away elated with a whole new life ahead, free from their former limitations and problems. This was accomplished with a minimum of time, utmost simplicity, maximum efficiency, and little cost.

From time to time I have been overwhelmed by frustration because of the refusal of orthodox fields to accept much-needed change in the healing field.

They are still burning witches in their own modern way. The orthodox mind condemns anything it doesn't understand. One would think that the many advances in technology in recent years would bring about a wholesome willingness to examine more closely any startling new discoveries in the healing field and allow them to be proven to their satisfaction. Despite all the tremendous research and sophisticated medication in the medical field, procedures have become odious, undesirable, fraught with multiple harmful side effects, and extremely costly.

Public reports are revealing that there is a substantial increase in sickness while the doctors admit they do not know the cause or correction of many of the crippling, and "incurable" diseases. This leads us to conclude that they may be doing something wrong.

Since I am willing and able to prove this work superior to anything in the healing field, it should be tested to its full capacities and, if it stands the test, be universally accepted and used for the benefit of the masses. One of the greatest humanitarian acts is to relieve pain and suffering.

It is time for the healing professions, and the laws which they have lobbied into existence, to change — to respect and realize that the needs and rights of the individual are more important than the ego of the doctor or the power of the law. I feel it is only fair and just that **each individual should have the right to make his own choice of healing method.**

In the past, the sick and the suffering had no place else to turn for relief or a cure. Now there is another method — and it should be given the same legal acceptability and respectability as those which have so abundantly demonstrated their inability to heal, but which have had the power to control the type of healing the public might choose.

It is of utmost importance that the sick and ailing be allowed to use a system of healing that has a long and consistent history of healing, completely free from faulty and costly errors. This system of automatic precision allows for no margin or personal mistakes. It is a system where trial and error is never present. So far, no other system has been able to produce anything approximating the past and present results of this system.

> *To many people, God seems so far away;*
> *If so — who did the moving?*

FROM PAGE ONE

73,000 elderly die yearly from drug error, reaction, study says

By Nancy Weaver
Bee Staff Writer

Each year in this country, 73,000 elderly die from adverse drug reactions or medication errors.

In California, medication problems send an estimated 180,000 people to the hospital each year, and that health care costs the state more than $500 million, said Betty Yee of the State Senate Office of Research.

"Every year, more seniors die of medication, not of a disease but adverse medication reaction, than all the people who died in Vietnam," said Kathy Borgan, of the Chemical Dependency Center for Women in Sacramento.

Because the elderly take an estimated 30 percent of all prescribed drugs and 70 percent of all over-the-counter medications, they experience more problems with their usage, according to experts in elderly health care.

Often suffering from multiple health problems, an older person may be taking several medications prescribed by more than one doctor and may not be aware of how they conflict, said Borgan, who works with the senior medication education program.

Medications often have a stronger effect on an elderly person than on a younger patient and the prescribing doctor may not be aware of that difference, she said.

For example, some medications may linger in the body longer because the liver functions of an elderly person cannot work as quickly to process out the drugs, said Borgan, who speaks to senior citizens groups on drug usage.

The mixture of over-the-counter drugs can contribute to problems with a prescription. And, increasingly, older people are sharing pills, using outdated drugs or substituting medications because prescriptions are so expensive.

"Modern medicine makes it possible for the elderly to live richer lives than we ever imagined. But when medicines don't match what they need, then it becomes a menace," said Betty Brill, acting chairwoman of the Sacramento chapter of the California Medication Education Coalition.

Brill urges all patients to ask doctors to explain potential side effects or other warnings. Family members who notice a change in behavior or other possible effects of medication problems should consult a doctor.

Gardis Mundt, a member of Families of Overmedicated Elderly which is educating people about medication uses, said her mother was nearly fitted for a hearing aid until she discovered that her hearing loss was only a temporary side effect of her medication.

Her mother was waiting for Mundt to pick her up for her doctor's appointment when she read the fine print on the medication sample bottle given to her by her doctor. The sample bottle specified potential hearing loss as a side effect.

"She quit taking the medication and she didn't need the hearing aid," said Mundt. She said her mother's doctor hadn't cautioned her of the side effects.

The California Pharmacists Association is sponsoring a "brown bag" program for member pharmacists to screen an elderly person's prescriptions for problems such as dangerous drug interactions or outdated medications.

Elderly people are urged to throw all the drugs from their medicine cabinet into a brown paper bag and have them examined by a pharmacist participating in various screening programs being held at different times. For more information, call the association at 1-800-444-3851.

The use of sedatives and mind-altering medications by elderly people in their own homes also is a growing problem. Borgan said senior citizens in this country also take 40 percent of all prescribed antipsychotic or tranquilizing medications such as Valium, Haldol and Mellaril.

Borgan said such medications often help a person survive the loss of a spouse or friends but that they must be used with caution.

"That generation has that magic pill formula. They're ready to take medications, too eager to take them," said Morgan. "Part of the problem is that they're kind on innocent in some cases. They're being poisoned."

149

Relieve Tension and Promote Circulation with
RELAX-A-ROLLER

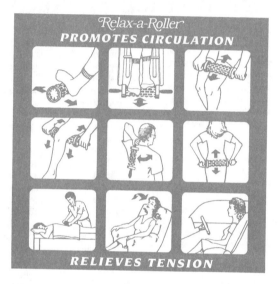

The Relax-a-Roller is a foot and body massager designed to create a reflex or pressure point massage similar to Vita-Flex or Reflexology. It is recommended by Chiropractors, Natruropaths and Reflexologists. An invigorating massage is accomplished by its unique design of pyramidal points which effectively break up tension. With just a few minutes of use tensions, drowsiness, weariness and pain disappear.

Originally created by Stanley Burroughs
and now manufactured by Vita-Gem Enterprises

The Relax-a-Roller can be ordered through Burrough's Books for $20.00 per unit plus $4.00 for shipping. Please add taxes where applicable.

Burroughs Books
3702 S. Virginia St. Ste. # G-12 Box 346 Reno, NV 89502-6030
Fax # 1-775-972-4899

LIFETIME WARRANTY

Enhance the Healing
with the **VITA-FLEX** video

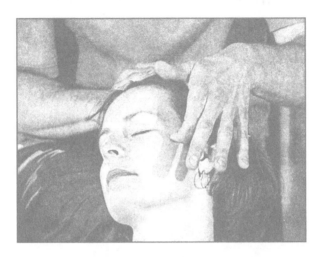

Vita-Flex is the ancient Tibetan massage technique that was rediscovered by Stanley Burroughs in the late 1920's. This unique technique has made Vita-Flex one of the most comprehensive, effective pressure or reflexive point massage in practice today.

The Vita-Flex video is a step by step instructional demonstration of the proper Vita-Flex technique and its application to specific areas of the body. Then a full Vita-Flex treatment is presented in three segments; Hands and Feet, Back and Shoulders and Head and Face including the Atlas Adjustment.

With this 75 minute video anyone can learn the proper Vita-Flex technique!

**Inquire about the amazing
miracle soap products from:**

**Burroughs Books
3702 S. Virginia St.
Ste. # G-12 Box 346
Reno, NV 89502-6030
Fax # 1-775-972-4899**

Notes

Notes